Praise for V

"*Breanne is a bright light that shines in this world, illuminating the way to a better life. She does her magic all with a wink and a smile, making it effortless and fun.*"

- Dr. Marisol Teijeiro, ND, AKA Queen of Thrones

"*If your goal is to feel good and look good,* Wild and Free *is a must-read! Why accept a life filled with digestive issues (disaster pants!), insidious weight gain, and crazy hormones when you have this incredible resource at your fingertips? Breanne clearly describes hormonal imbalances and leaky gut so you will feel educated and empower to become your own health advocate.*"

- Kate Jaramillo, creator of the Ketogenic Living Certification program

"*Breanne is a most trusted colleague and friend of mine. Her book is a must-have resource for anyone struggling to sort out the often times confusing world of alternative medicine. This book will give you the ability to skillfully leverage dietary and lifestyle choices if you are seeking balanced hormones, increased energy, and overall body confidence.*"

- Lisa Marie Holmes, Herbalist and Founder of Wild One Herbs

"*Inspirational and life changing. Dr. Breanne Kallonen brings you a functional and back to basics approach that will give you the tools to be healthy for a lifetime.*"

- Dr. Robin Walsh, ND

"*Dr. Breanne is a true gift to women and medicine. Her genius is sharing complex medical information as straightforward, easy to understand solutions to women's health struggles. This book is a gem — thank you Dr. Breanne for inspiring your patients and your colleagues.*"

- Dr. Glenna Calder, ND

Wild and Free

Get Back the Body You Love Naturally

Dr. Breanne Kallonen, ND

This book is not intended as a substitute for medical advice. Please consult your medical professional before making any changes to your health and fitness routine or your diet. The author and publisher disclaim any liability or loss, personal or otherwise, that might result from the information and plans provided in this book.

DEDICATION

The completion of this undertaking would not have occurred without the help of so many people. I would like to express my deepest gratitude to my patients and Wild Side Wellness tribe who have put faith in their own innate ability to heal. Without your stories and determination to discovering your own root cause this book would not be possible.

Thank you to my family and friends who have supported me and been there through thick and thin. To my colleagues and mentors thank you for continuing to inspire and create impact on a global scale; continue to share your work, passion, and beliefs and most importantly, never lose sight of the importance of the work we do.

CONTENTS

Introduction   1

1   Why You Need This Book   5

2   Love Your Liver   9

3   The Adrenals   20

4   Thyroid   31

5   Sex Hormones   42

6   Fat Hormones   70

7   Brain Hormones   75

8   Mind Your Mitochondria   86

9   Digestion and Gut Health   93

10   Blood Sugar, Insulin Resistance, and Glucagon   104

11   Genetics   115

12   Sleep   126

13   Nutrition   130

14   Workouts   144

15   Autoimmunity   157

16   Mindset   156

Appendix: Supplements   179

Additional Resources   182

INTRODUCTION

"I have found that if you love life, life will love you back"
-Arthur Rubinstein

CAN YOU IMAGINE BEING SO TIRED YOU ARE AFRAID TO FALL ASLEEP DRIVING, SO FOGGY YOUR HEAD IS BUZZING WITH CONFUSION? Can you image suffering from food cravings so badly that they felt like you had lost all control? Can you imagine gaining weight despite eating the same way, losing hair, and having menstrual cycles that are all over the map? Well, that was me and my story is no different than many of the clients I work with.

I am a high achieving woman. I want more; I want it all. I want to feel good, I want to look good, and I want to achieve greatness. I want to be a leader for my family and for my community. This is what I want. My story is that I started young. I started my family my business and earned my Doctor of Naturopathy Degree by age 25 and I kept wanting more. But the more I pushed, the more my body rebelled.

My first sign was fatigue. I went to my doctor to investigate further into why I was so tired. I was told I was anemic with extremely low iron levels. My thyroid was "normal," but of course at the time I did not receive proper testing (more on that in the upcoming/thyroid chapters). Because my weight appeared "normal," my doctor did not think of looking deeper into hypothyroidism despite having every symptom including fatigue, cold intolerance, hair loss, irregular cycles, constipation, and a thyroid any untrained individual could feel.

After my appointment, my doctor recommended that I take iron, and that was the end of it. My gut knew there was more going on because at the time I was breastfeeding and not menstruating and also consuming a decent amount of red meat. Nevertheless, I accepted my diagnosis as anemia and "too much" going on.

In order to get any ounce of energy I could, I became addicted to caffeine, sugar and fatty foods. I craved them so badly that I felt completely out of control. After meals, I would feel exhausted and anxious. The more sugar I ate, the more addicted I became. My skin started to break out and my constipation and bloating got worse. As a Naturopathic Doctor, I knew the sugary processed treats were wreaking havoc on my hormones, but with the fatigue, constant hunger, and extreme cravings, I felt like I could not stop.

The second sign was very troublesome and something I hid and compensated for a long time. Growing up it was quite evident that I had a photographic memory. I would memorize the eye chart prior to being tested to avoid having to get glasses. I would remember virtually everything I read, and school came very easily for me. I was always told how "smart" I was and I embodied that as my identity.

As I approached the time to study for my Naturopathic Physician Licensing Examination (NPLEX), I started to forget details. I could no longer remember people's names, and I was having extreme difficulty staying on task. I would purchase calendar after calendar and sticky notes filled my desktop and home. I was so embarrassed because I truly did not recognize the slow, clumsy person I had become. I vividly remember one day looking at my computer screen and I had at least 20 different browser tabs open. I was in tears overwhelmed and the confusion was overcoming me because my brain function was slowing down like the rest of me.

The last major wake up call for me was my mood. Words were flying out of my mouth before I could grab them. I was impatient, frustrated, and certainly not myself, especially around my children. I did not recognize my behaviour. How I was acting wasn't "me," and it was certainly not something I was comfortable with.

Equipped with all the tools and resources, I finally ditched all excuses and underwent a thorough investigation of conventional and functional medicine laboratory tests. My suspicion was confirmed: I had virtually every hormone imbalance in the book including insulin resistance, hypothyroidism, high cortisol, estrogen dominance, and low progesterone and DHEA, to name a few. As the demands on me through my twenties continued to evolve, so did the complexity of my hormonal havoc. Thank goodness I possess the tools, education, resources, and ability to not only identify these underlying issues but also reverse them to a state of balance. Through diet, lifestyle, supplements, and specific compounded thyroid medication, I was able to heal my hormones and have a much clearer view of the big picture.

Part of my story is wanting to have it all, be it all, and do it all. I was hustling hard, running at a million miles per minute and juggling multiple balls at once. It worked for a while and it got me through med school, but eventually those balls started to drop. Chances are if you have picked up this book, yours are too. As women, we often count our defeats and losses rather than celebrating our wins. We focus on the negative and get entangled in our *current problem or diagnosis* instead of focusing on our *desired outcome*. In order to correct and heal hormone imbalances, the very first thing you must do is undergo a paradigm shift in order to gain a new perspective. The foundation I want to present to you now is rooted in questions such as: what makes us happy, optimistic, and thrive, and what enhances our wellbeing? By focusing on having fun every day and what makes life worth living, we automatically make the first shift into allowing our body, mind, and spirit to become transformed.

We live in an all-or-nothing society that has become accustomed to immediate satisfaction. In a day of modern technology, multitasking, and impatience, I invite you to accept yourself where you are at today. Accept that your healing journey is uniquely your own and that you are aiming for progress, not perfection. I invite you to be okay with slow incremental improvements while still recognizing areas in which you can improve upon. Allow yourself the grace to be okay with the path you are currently on and be open to even better experiences to come. Things can be better and they will be. Let's do this.

What Kind of Doctor Am I?

I am a Naturopathic Doctor (ND). *Naturopathic Medicine* is an evidence-based system that uses natural therapies and methods to restore health and wellness, optimize health and prevent disease. The focus I take is treating the underlying cause rather than the symptoms. In addition, I take a functional medicine approach and aim to optimize functioning of the body and its organs, supporting all organ systems using holistic or alternative medicine. Treatments I promote in my practice include diet, lifestyle, exercise, herbs, supplements, avoidance of toxins/chemicals, reduction of stress and supporting detoxification.

CHAPTER 1

Why You Need This Book

YOU DO YOUR BEST TO HAVE IT ALL...BUT YOU'RE SACRIFICING YOURSELF AND YOUR HEALTH. As you hustle and push through the tough stuff, no matter what, that mentality becomes your reality and perpetuates sympathetic overwhelm aka burnout.

Unfortunately, it doesn't stop there. Burnout is just the beginning...next comes, exhaustion, brain fog, irritability, thyroid conditions, hormone imbalances, chronic fatigue syndrome, autoimmune disease and more.

This was my reality, and it's the story I hear from so many of my patients. My hope it that by the end of this book you obtain the tools and feel empowered to start your journey either towards healing or health optimization. To get started, let's review some of the most common signs and symptoms of hormone imbalances.

Are Your Symptoms Signs of Hormonal Imbalance?

Do any of these symptoms sound familiar?

- Weight gain or inability to lose weight
- Anxiety & depression
- PMS
- Fatigue
- Low libido
- Cold intolerance
- Hair loss
- Insomnia
- Painful periods, or clotting
- Difficulty falling asleep or staying asleep
- Feeling stressed or overwhelmed
- Irritable mood
- Blood sugar imbalances
- Irregular menstrual cycles
- Fibrocystic breasts
- PCOS, endometriosis, and/or fibroids
- Joint pain and muscle aches

If you can identify with some or many of the symptoms listed above, you may be experiencing hormone imbalance. The key to healthy hormones is to support the whole body, with a special focus on the liver, gut, ovaries, adrenals, and thyroid. A multi-system approach, like the one described in this book, is the best way to overcome this large suite of symptoms. Ideally, your solution should integrate diet, lifestyle, laboratory testing, physical examination, stress management, and sleep. That's exactly what I'll teach you to do if you keep reading.

If your hormones are out of whack, you're not alone. Imbalances of hormones such as thyroid hormones, DHEA, cortisol, growth hormone, insulin, testosterone, progesterone and estrogen are quite common and often difficult to correct.

Hormone imbalances can present themselves in some interesting ways. Some signs your system is out of whack are feeling tired throughout the day, difficulties concentrating or brain fog, inability to lose weight, and inexplicably feeling down.

Things can get even more complicated for women because our hormones naturally fluctuate monthly. Our menstrual cycles are actually very complex and must be orchestrated precisely so we can feel our best. Lifestyle factors such as eating inflammatory foods or not getting enough sleep can have profound impacts on our hormone levels. I know! It's kind of a bummer, but luckily there are simple strategies you can implement to begin getting your hormones back on track.

Estrogen and progesterone are the main female sex hormones, although women do have varying levels of testosterone. Typically, women have lower testosterone levels than men, but levels can be raised by conditions such as PCOS. When estrogen and progesterone are out of balance, they are rarely the only ones. In fact, your hormonal imbalance may stem from issues with your thyroid, adrenals, liver, gut, and diet, and from lifestyle factors.

Because you are a whole person and every part of you is connected, I rarely if ever, only address female sex hormones when patients come see me looking to restore balance.

Your liver, gut, ovaries, thyroid and adrenals all need to be functioning optimally together to restore hormone balance. Specifically, you can think of the ovaries, adrenals, and thyroid as a three-legged stool. If one leg is weak or missing, the stool is not strong, and the whole system risks collapsing. In addition, the liver and gut are foundational; if you have an uneven floor, your stool risks collapsing.

How to Find Hormonal Balance

To start to find hormonal imbalances, you need to start listening to your body. Trust the signals it's sending to you. You know your body better than anyone, and you can tell when something's not right. To balance your hormones, you need to trust your gut! So often we ignore what our bodies are telling us.

The first step in achieving hormonal balance, boosting your energy, healing disease, and reducing fat stores is to start with building a strong foundation. The focus needs to be on nourishing your body with REAL foods, removing toxins and inflammation while adding minerals and vitamins to correct deficiencies. This will put your body into a relaxed, healing state. By focusing on strengthening any areas of deficiencies, you are giving your body the best chance to use its natural processes to promote healing and repair.

The interventions in the following chapters are lifestyle changes that can be potentially lifesaving for you. If you are looking for a quick fix or magic unicorn pill, I would suggest you stop reading. These lifestyle changes will require commitment and additional effort, as well as spending money on quality foods and supplements. In my opinion, this is a small price to pay in order to live longer, experience more, and take more vacations. I am not in the business to save people money on their mortgages; I am here to preserve health and reverse disease. The great news is that most people feel significantly better in a relatively short amount of time when they implement these lifestyle changes. Some people, just by supporting their body's own healing abilities, will reverse symptoms and regain a more energized, balanced life.

CHAPTER TWO

Love Your Liver

Welcome to the first phase of your healing journey. In this chapter you will kickstart your body's natural healing process by removing hidden toxins from your everyday life and support your liver to detoxify hormones and toxins that are residing within you. Many symptoms clients come to me with can be linked to an impaired detoxification system. Often these people report the most significant improvements in how they feel when their detoxification pathways become more efficient. Along with your lungs, skin, and kidneys, the liver plays a critical role in detoxification and will be what we are targeting first.

The world we live in today is filled with an unprecedented number of toxins. The air we breathe, the water we drink, the foods we eat, and the lotions and sprays we slather on our skin all are constantly putting our system into overload. If your body's natural detoxification systems are in any way impaired due to genetics, nutrient deficiencies, stress, inflammation, or simply from being overburdened, you are going to struggle to handle toxins. Being exposed to the quantity of toxins in our environment coupled with a genetic predisposition may be the perfect storm of vulnerabilities to spark autoimmune disease and endocrine imbalances.

The liver is the main organ of detoxification along with the skin, kidneys, and lungs. Liver dysfunction can contribute to digestive issues, inability to convert inactive thyroid hormone (T4) to active thyroid hormone (T3), skin breakouts, sensitivities, insulin resistance, fatigue, and more. The goal of the liver support protocol you'll find in this chapter is to make your body more resilient to the toxic burden you face on a daily basis.

Signs and Symptoms of Toxicity

Acne
Anger, irritability, frustration, aggression
Arthritis
Asthma, bronchitis
Bags or dark circles under eyes
Bad breath
Belching or passing gas
Binge eating or drinking
Bloating
Blurred or tunnel vision
Brain fog
Canker sores
Chest congestion
Chest pain
Chronic coughing
Compulsive eating
Confusion, poor comprehension
Constipation
Craving certain foods
Depression
Diarrhea
Difficulty breathing
Difficulty in making decisions
Digestive problems
Dizziness
Drainage from the ear, itchy ears
Ear aches, ear infections
Eczema
Emotional dysregulation

Excessive mucus
Excessive sweating
Excessive weight
Faintness
Fatigue, feeling sluggish
Feeling weak or tired
Food sensitivities
Flushing or hot flashes
Frequent illnesses
Frequent or urgent urination
Gagging, frequent need to clear throat
Genital itching or discharge
Hair loss
Hay fever
Headaches
Heartburn
Hives, rashes, or dry skin
Hormonal imbalances
Hyperactivity
Insomnia
Intestinal or stomach pain
Irregular or skipped heartbeat
Itchy ears
Learning disabilities
Mood swings
Multiple chemical sensitivities
Nausea or vomiting
Near or farsightedness
One or more autoimmune diseases
Pain or aches in joints
Pain or aches in muscles
Poor concentration
Poor memory
Poor physical coordination
Rapid or pounding heartbeat
Restlessness
Ringing in ears, hearing loss
Sensitivity to medications and supplements
Shortness of breath

Sinus problems
Slurred speech
Sneezing attacks
Sore throat, hoarseness, loss of voice
Stiffness or limitation of movement
Stuffy nose
Stuttering or stammering
Swollen, reddened or sticky eyelids
Swollen or discoloured tongue, gums, lips
Underweight
Unexplained weakness
Water retention
Watery, itchy eyes

Do any of these symptoms sound familiar? If you're like the majority of my patients, they do. And, because your liver plays such a critical and crucial role in your health, you should begin your journey to balance your hormones by supporting the natural functions of your liver.

Here are the ways you should support your liver:

1. Remove and reduce exposure to toxins and potentially triggering foods
2. Add in healing foods - cruciferous vegetables and adequate protein
3. Correct nutrient deficiencies
4. Support detox pathways - liver, bowel, skin, lungs, kidneys
5. Supplement smartly

We will address these strategies in greater detail throughout this chapter and the rest of the book.

Phases of Liver Detoxification

The liver's detoxification processes can be broken down into two phases: phase 1 and phase 2. You'll learn more about these two phases, as well as what happens to estrogen as it goes through liver detoxification. Many other compounds are processed in a similar way. As you learn about these processes, you'll gain a better understanding of how your liver affects the hormones in your body, and your health as a whole.

In phase 1 detox, estrogen produced by the ovaries (estradiol) is covered into a "harmful" intermediate called estrone. A potentially harmful intermediate is common for phase 1, which is why it is so important for phase 1 and phase 2 to be balanced. You might think that the solution would be to slow down or stop phase 1 if it produces that dangerous intermediate. But, it is important that phase 1 does not slow down, because if it does, hormone imbalances arise. A great way to support phase 1 detox is to consume 3,3'-Diindolylmethane (DIM), and phytonutrients derived from cruciferous vegetables such as cauliflower, broccoli, Brussels sprouts, and cabbage.

Phase 2 detox is also referred to as the conjugation pathway. In this phase, the liver adds additional compounds like amino acids and nutrients to toxic chemicals and hormones that have already been processed by phase 1. Adding the compounds to the toxic chemicals renders them harmless. This step makes the substances water-soluble, allowing them to be easily excreted and removed by the body through the urine or stool.

Efficient phase 2 detoxification requires methylation, which in turn requires methyl groups to complete the process. In order for the liver to have adequate supply of methyl groups, which your body receives from an optimal intake of vitamins B6, B12 and B9. Another process in phase 2 requires sulfur-containing amino acids like glycine, glutamine, and choline. In this step, sulfur groups are added to hormones such as estrogen so they can be easily excreted. Luckily, these sulfur compounds are found in foods such as egg yolks, animal proteins, garlic, onions, and Brussels sprouts.

After hormones such as estrogen are processed in the liver, they make their way to the intestines for removal. But, the process hits a roadblock if unhealthy bacteria are abundant in the intestine. This collection of bacteria that impacts estrogen levels is known as the estrobolome.

In a healthy person, estrogens are further processed for removal via a process called glucuronidation. When unhealthy, abnormal bacteria are present in large numbers, glucuronidation is stopped. These bacteria can actually produce an enzyme that alters the estrogen molecules, allowing them to be reabsorbed into the bloodstream. The excess estrogen in the blood contributes to estrogen dominance.

Calcium-D-glucarate, a supplement I use often, can render the enzyme inactive and prevent the buildup of excess estrogen. Supplementing with a probiotic can also help good bacteria outnumber and thus outcompete the bad bacteria.

Lastly, glutathione conjugation can assist in removal of hormones like estrogen through phase 2 detoxification. It is also a sulfur-containing molecule that is added to estrogen for easy removal. I have many of my patients supplement with liposomal glutathione or NAC (N-acetyl cysteine), as well as consume foods like whey protein (if not sensitive), walnuts, asparagus, and sulfur-rich foods. It is also important that you ensure your nutrient status is optimized, because the lack of nutrients and amino acids may reduce glutathione levels.

Our Toxic Environment

One of the top reasons why I believe we suffer from chronic disease is our exposure to toxic industrial chemicals in our air, water, food, and household and personal products. It really has gotten out of control. Our bodies are great at detoxifying and do it effortlessly, but we were never meant to carry such a large toxic burden. There are formaldehyde fumes in furniture, chloride and fluoride in our water, electromagnetic fields from the gadgets in our homes, BPA in sales receipts, chemicals in factory-farmed food, herbicides and pesticides in our food and environment, perfluorinated compounds (PFCs) in carpet and fluorescent lights, and thousands of exposures to plastics every day. With the level of toxin exposure, it is no wonder our genes, hormones, energy levels, and waistlines are struggling.

This is why you should eat organic when possible, or at least avoid the dirty dozen (more info at www.ewg.org). You should also filter your water, avoid chemical-laden products, and when you clean our home, use natural cleaners like vinegar, baking soda, and lemon essential oil. For information on products I personally use to detox, check out the appendix at the back of this book.

Xenoestrogens

Just one example of toxins in our environment are xenoestrogens. These compounds are found in and throughout our environment. They're particularly dangerous because they imitate estrogens in our bodies. Having exposure to environmental estrogens is a contributor to estrogen dominance. That exposure also overburdens the liver's detoxification processes.

Signs of estrogen dominance include PMS, weight gain, blood clots, heavy periods, fibrocystic breasts, and endometriosis, as well as an increased risk for estrogen-related cancers. Estrogen also impacts thyroid hormone by reducing the conversion of inactive T4 to active T3, blocking the uptake of thyroid hormone, and by increasing thyroid binding globulin (TBG). When TBG is increased, it binds to more thyroid hormone and prevents it from binding to thyroid receptors on cells and produces hypothyroid symptoms. [1] And, that's all on top of the effects that an estrogen-based birth control pill causes.

---

[1] Santin, Ana Paula, and Tania Weber Furlanetto. "Role of estrogen in thyroid function and growth regulation." Journal of Thyroid Research 2011 (2011)

Halogens

Halogens are a group of elements in the periodic table that include bromide, chloride and fluoride, as well as iodine. Because bromide, chloride, and fluoride are structurally similar to iodine, they may take up receptor sites on the thyroid gland and create thyroid imbalances and disturbances. My recommendation would be to avoid chemicals with high levels of these elements at all cost. Sources of halogens include water, baked goods, plastics, pesticides, fire retardants, pools, soda, and medications

How to Love on Your Liver

Your body is an amazingly complex system, working day in and day out to eliminate toxins and excess hormones. In addition, your body is simultaneously breaking down and absorbing the food you eat into nutrients to fuel each and every cell. In order to support your body, you need your detox organs to be in tip-top shape, and at the centre of detoxification is your liver.

Our natural detoxification pathways help conjugate and clear exogenous chemicals, toxins, hormones, and byproducts of cellular processes. The body avoids a buildup of potentially harmful toxins and helps us to feel our best by having a system of multiple organs of elimination. When detoxification and elimination pathways are functioning properly, we produce hormones and neurotransmitters in an optimal way.

But here's where we run into trouble. Our environment is full of toxins, endocrine-disrupting chemicals, carcinogens, pesticides, and flame retardants (to just name a few) and we're chronically stressed. All of these factors can quickly knock hormones levels out of whack and leave you feeling like anything but yourself. When your hormones are imbalanced, your mood, menstrual cycle, energy, weight, complexion, bowels, etc. are affected.

Plus, hormone balance is necessary for fertility. If you are trying to get pregnant, we must get your sex hormones to the right levels in your body and working together to allow for conception and to support a healthy pregnancy. So, if you are trying to conceive, natural detoxification is one technique you may want to consider.

This simple and easy at-home technique helps to support your liver, and bowels to encourage detoxification and waste elimination. In addition to the home detox tool I share below, focus on consuming liver-loving foods, reducing stress, and getting adequate sleep.

Home Detox Tool: Castor Oil Packs

Castor oil is made from the castor bean and has been used historically for a variety of ailments, internally and externally. Please do not take castor oil internally unless you have consulted with your doctor. (Your family, friends, roommates, and toilet will thank you.) Internally, castor oil stimulates the bowels and increases circulation. From personal experience, it causes extreme cramping and explosive diarrhea — proceed with caution!

Topically, castor oil packs can be placed over the abdomen to enhance liver function, stimulate the healthy flow of lymph fluid, decrease inflammation, and help treat chronic constipation.

Castor Oil Packs for Liver Detoxification

Instructions:

1. Purchase castor oil, preferably oil that has been stored in a dark glass container. I use the Queen of Thrones Castor Oil Packs created by my amazing colleague and friend Dr. Marisol, ND, AKA the Queen of Thrones.
2. Every night before bed, apply castor oil from your midsection (hip bone to lower ribs). Rub in a clockwise direction. *Note: castor oil will darken and stain fabric over time.
3. Apply a piece of flannel, old towel, or old shirt over your

midsection.

4. You can apply heat or skip it, whatever is convenient.
5. Ideally, you should use this time to relax, meditate, or read.
6. Go to bed and have a great sleep.
7. Repeat the following night.

Castor oil packs are just as simple as that. They increase circulation, stimulate the bowels, and support liver detoxification. This is just one of the many natural ways to improve hormone health and create an abundance of happiness, energy, and strength.

In addition to castor oil packs, you should consider the following lifestyle changes as your liver is often at the root of hormone imbalances:

- Eat quality protein.
- Eat plenty of garlic and onions.
- Take a B vitamin complex.
- Eat a minimum of three cups of cruciferous vegetables weekly.
- Don't smoke and keep alcohol to a minimum (fewer than four drinks per week).
- Eat only organic meats and dairy, and follow the Environmental Working Group Clean 15 and Dirty Dozen (website info located in the additional resources section)
- Use natural household cleaners, cosmetics, and body products. As women, we apply more than 15 different products to our bodies before we even leave the house in the morning. Many of these products are made using a dozen or more chemicals. There are many fantastic natural cosmetics available to us now.
- Avoid unnecessary medications.
- Correct nutritional deficiencies — you cannot detox when you are deficient in cofactors.
- Support detox pathways — other than your liver, the bowel, skin, lungs, and kidneys are responsible for removing toxins.

Ensure that you are sweating daily, consider using saunas, and drink plenty of clean water.

- Make sure your bowels are moving every day — at least once! If you're constipated, consider taking between 300 mg and 600 mg of magnesium bisglycinate every night, and take 1-3 tablespoons of a fibre source in the AM and PM to get things going.
- Drink a bitter tonic twice daily for one week. To make your own spring liver tonic/cleanse, try this bitters drink:

    Use 1/4 teaspoons each of the following herbal tinctures: dandelion root, burdock root, artichoke, sarsaparilla root, and ginger root.

A trusted botanical brand is Wild One Herbals created by my colleague and friend Lisa Holmes.

CHAPTER THREE

The Adrenals

LET ME ASK YOU: DO YOU RESONATE WITH ANY OF THESE SYMPTOMS?

You are tired…or more like exhausted.
You can't sleep.
You frequently become sick.
You have gained extra weight, but no matter how little you eat or how much you exercise, the pounds don't seem to budge.
You can't imagine going about your day without coffee.
You regularly feel unmotivated, not yourself, or even overwhelmed at times.

If you have experienced one or many of the symptoms on that list, you are in good company…I've personally experienced all of these symptoms and have helped plenty of women just like you!

I hear about women experiencing these symptoms all the time, whether they're my patients, my friends, or simply other women in my network. Many women who come to me have hit a health and fitness plateau. They are completely burnt out and have tried everything to lose weight. I frequently see new clients who have been consistently working out, even six or seven times per week, but who are not seeing results.

Many of my clients have been conditioned to eat breakfast as soon as they wake up to get their metabolism "going." They also are eating several small meals per day, which is constantly spiking their insulin levels. They do intense workouts, which are combined with overwhelming everyday stress. That physical and mental stress have completely thrown their cortisol levels out of whack. To make matters worse, many women come to me who are significantly under eating for the workouts they are doing.

The overall result is flattened energy levels, feeling anxious, often feeling a bit depressed, and the inability to lose fat around the midsection. These symptoms may be due to hypothyroidism or adrenal fatigue induced by harmful (but well-intended) diet and exercise habits. We'll focus on the thyroid and hypothyroidism in the next chapter; for now, I'd like to turn your attention to your adrenal glands.

All About Adrenals

You have two walnut-sized adrenal glands that sit on top of each of your kidneys. Tiny and mighty, these glands secrete a variety of different hormones and chemicals necessary for survival. The two we will focus on in this book are adrenaline (epinephrine) and cortisol. Together they regulate your blood sugar, level of inflammation, ability to fight infection, fat storage, energy, sex drive, hormone cycles, and fertility. They also play a critical role in providing you with fuel to escape a dangerous situation.

Adrenaline

When you are in a stressful situation, real or perceived, your body responds to the threat by producing adrenaline. This increases your heart rate and moves blood away from digestive organs to your muscles, allowing you to fight if needed. Your respiratory system will dilate to allow for more oxygen to be brought in, your blood pressure rises, your immune system mobilizes its defenses, your pupils dilate, and you are in a state of hyper vigilance (meaning you are alert and sensitive to everything).

In the short term, adrenaline is a rush — it keeps you on the edge of your seat in a scary movie or provides the thrill of a rollercoaster ride. But, when it becomes activated too often, it can leave you feeling wired, always on edge, and can negatively affect your heart and elevate blood pressure, to name just a few symptoms.

Cortisol

Cortisol is your stress hormone. When you are stressed, your body releases cortisol and catecholamines. Your body cannot tell the difference between stress from work or kids or a real life-and-death situation. Over time, elevated cortisol will cause you to store fat around your midsection. It will also increase your appetite and cravings for sugary, fatty foods.

After being exposed to a stressor, your brain senses that you are in danger, and it sends the signals to your adrenals to produce and release cortisol within minutes. Cortisol frees up glucose to provide extra energy to run or fight the danger. Insulin is released in response to the elevated blood sugar, as too much sugar causes inflammation and damage. Cortisol kicks your immune system into full gear, amping up protective boundaries against infections. In addition, cortisol dramatically alters not only the integrity of your gut, but also the microbiome that occupies it. Your brain also gets affected and turns into more of an autopilot mode rather than using willpower and higher critical thinking abilities.

Over time, elevated cortisol becomes an issue and your body pays the price. The result is chronically high blood pressure, high blood sugar, and even insulin resistance when your pancreas becomes too fatigued to keep producing extra insulin. You begin to store weight around the middle, cholesterol builds, and you experience relentless sugar, fat, carb, or salt cravings. You always feel on edge due to adrenaline, which prevents you from falling asleep and alters your sleep-wake cycle.

Your immune system becomes so imbalanced that you can eventually develop an autoimmune condition. Most often, the autoimmune condition affects the thyroid due to the impact cortisol has on thyroid function. When this happens, the overstimulated and wired feeling you once felt turns into fatigue or extreme exhaustion.

The New Understanding of HPA Axis Dysfunction

Since beginning my practice, I have moved away from using the term "adrenal fatigue." Instead, I refer to the phenomenon as hypothalamic-pituitary adrenal (HPA) axis dysfunction, and here is why. There is a misconception that the adrenal glands give out, and this simply is just not true. Unlike the ovaries which stop functioning during menopause, the adrenals do not simply stop making cortisol. This is just not true.

What actually happens is that we are assaulted by stressors all day, whether it is inside of us (i.e. pain, inflammation, blood sugar issues) or outside of us (i.e. stress, chemicals in our environment, toxic thoughts). The brain perceives these stimuli and tells the adrenals to put out cortisol. If the brain doesn't send the right signals, the adrenal glands will not function properly. So, it is not the lack of adrenal function, but rather the lack of appropriate signalling from the brain that results in the changes in symptoms and values we see when we test hormone levels.

In addition, I want to clarify that the symptoms you are experiencing are real. When you have hypothalamic-pituitary-adrenal dysfunction, you absolutely feel fatigued, exhausted, and unlike yourself, and I 100% believe you and I believe that you are experiencing these symptoms.

The Cortisol Awakening Response (CAR)

What is the cortisol awakening response (CAR) and how do we test it?

The cortisol awakening response is the ability of your brain to tell your adrenals, "You have to make cortisol first thing in the morning." The very second we open our eyes when we wake up, cortisol levels naturally begin to rise, doubling on average. Cortisol should spike up in the morning and follow a predictable pattern: 30 minutes after you wake up, we should see a sharp increase in cortisol. After 60 minutes, cortisol levels should hit their peak value for the day and begin to decline. Measuring this rise and fall of cortisol levels at waking can be used as a "mini stress-test." Some people do this really well, while others overshoot the moon, and some don't produce nearly enough cortisol.

A low or blunted CAR can be a result of:

- an underactive HPA axis
- excessive psychological burnout
- seasonal affective disorder (SAD)
- sleep apnea or poor sleep in general
- PTSD
- chronic fatigue and/or chronic pain.

A decreased CAR has also been associated with systemic hypertension, functional GI diseases, postpartum depression, and autoimmune diseases. Cortisol also plays a really important role in telling your thymus gland to kill cells tagged as autoimmune. When the CAR is disrupted, those autoimmune cells can escape. That's why so many people say their autoimmune symptoms are worse in the morning.

An elevated CAR can be a result of:

- an over-reactive HPA axis

- ongoing job-related stress (anticipatory stress for the day)
- blood sugar dysregulation
- pain (i.e. waking with painful joints or a migraine)
- general depression (not SAD)

A recent study[2] showed that neither the waking nor post-waking cortisol levels correlated to Major Depressive Disorder, but the CAR calculation (the difference between the two samples) did.

So, how do you test if you have a healthy CAR, or if it's low or elevated? A quick saturation of saliva swabs upon waking, and at 30 and 60 minutes after waking, provide what is required to assess a patient's cortisol awakening response. To see if this testing is appropriate for you, speak with a Functional Medicine Practitioner or Naturopathic Doctor. For more information on the testing visit https://dutchtest.com

The Androgens: DHEA and Testosterone

The androgens or "male hormones" androsterone, DHEA, and testosterone are often neglected in women's health, but they are critically important. While women do not produce as much of these hormones as men, having the appropriate levels of these hormones can be a game changer for mood, libido, fat loss, energy levels, and the prevention of premature aging.

Testosterone

In women, testosterone is produced by both the adrenals and the ovaries. This is why when you are under stress, testosterone

---

[2] Adam EK, Doane LD, Zinbarg RE, Mineka S, Craske MG, Gri th JW. Prospective prediction of major depressive disorder from cortisol awakening responses in adolescence. Psychoneuroendocrinology. 2010 Jul 35(6):921-31.

decreases—your adrenal glands are focusing more on producing cortisol to deal with the perceived stressor than sex hormones like testosterone that get you in the mood to reproduce.

In both sexes, low testosterone can lead to symptoms such as depression, obesity, heart disease, low libido, diminished motivation, loss of muscle mass, insomnia, fatigue, brain fog, and increased body fat. Taking into consideration your symptoms as well as results from laboratory testing can help determine if you need additional testosterone. Hormones are complex, and supplementing can be beneficial, but it does not come without risk. So, if you're considering supplementation, it makes good medical sense to have your levels tested. I would suggest looking at both free and total testosterone levels if you can.

Testosterone and Weight Loss

There is a win-win relationship between testosterone and weight loss. Research shows that testosterone increases weight loss, and weight loss increases testosterone. And, exercise increases both — even better! In a 2011 study from the American Diabetes Society, scientists showed that low testosterone was associated with obesity and metabolic syndrome, and it contributed to sexual dysfunction and cardiovascular disease risk.[3] So, if you've been struggling to lose weight, low testosterone may be part of the reason why. Luckily, there are ways to support your adrenal health and boost testosterone production naturally.

Increase Testosterone Naturally

If you suffer from low libido, fatigue, reduced muscle mass, low

---

[3] Wang, Christina, et al. "Low testosterone associated with obesity and the metabolic syndrome contributes to sexual dysfunction and cardiovascular disease risk in men with type 2 diabetes." Diabetes care 34.7 (2011): 1669-1675.

motivation, and brain fog and your labs indicate low testosterone, it is time to give yourself a boost. As with many of the other hormones, testosterone levels decline with age, increased stress, and higher body weight. But, you don't have to accept these symptoms as an inevitable part of aging. Let's examine some ways that you can increase the amount of testosterone your body produces naturally.

To boost your body's testosterone production, you may want to implement the following lifestyle habits:

- Sleeping the right amount for your body
- Exercise (both cardio and strength training)
- Having sex that includes orgasms
- Getting outside in the sun
- Practice daily self-care for stress relief

Lifestyle changes may seem unimportant, but they can make a big difference.

Dietary modifications to increase testosterone include consuming adequate protein, carbohydrates and fats. With the current ketogenic craze, carbs are getting a bad rap, but they are critical for maintaining thyroid and testosterone levels. In addition, complete carb restriction can be a stress on the body, increasing cortisol levels, which then further reduce testosterone levels. Carbohydrates especially after a workout are important to raise insulin, the anabolic hormone that helps to grow and maintain muscle mass. In the right amount, insulin preserves muscle mass and supplies your cells with the amino acids, glucose, and fatty acids needed to grow, heal, and repair.

Here are some supplements you might also consider adding to boost testosterone production:

- Tribulus (*Tribulus terrestris*) (aerial)
- Tongkat ali (*Eurycoma longifolia*) (root)
- DHEA (Dehydroepiandrosterone)
- Arginine

- Adrenal Support
- Detox — Excess estrogen is often associated with low testosterone. Detoxing assists with removing harmful estrogens.
- Bioidentical testosterone
- Zinc — A deficiency in zinc has been shown to lower LH (luteinizing hormone). Zinc also appears to reduce the aromatisation of testosterone to estrogen. Take 25-50 mg with food.

DHEA

DHEA (dehydroepiandrosteone) is a hormone that is produced primarily by the adrenal glands. It is very important because it serves as a precursor to the sex hormones estrogen and testosterone.

DHEA has been coined as the "anti-aging" hormone because it counteracts the negative effects of cortisol. DHEA can alter fat metabolism, fertility, sex drive, energy, and muscle mass. It also improves your brain health and the appearance of your skin. Furthermore, DHEA is known to impact the immune system, and low levels appear to be associated with autoimmune diseases.[4] DHEA has been shown to reduce antibodies and be protective for those with autoimmune disease. And, DHEA can also act like a natural anti-depressant by helping to improve your mood.

Like all the other hormones, the key is to maintain optimal levels in balance with all the other hormones. More is not better. Many women with androgen excess have a condition known as PCOS, or polycystic ovarian syndrome. This can lead to male pattern hair growth, irregular cycles, acne, and a deepening voice.

---

[4] Van Vollenhoven, Ronald F., Edgar G. Engleman, and James L. Mcguire. "Dehydroepiandrosterone in systemic lupus erythematosus." *Arthritis & Rheumatology* 38.12 (1995): 1826-1831.

Increase DHEA Naturally

Have orgasms — Oxytocin, the bonding or love hormone, has the ability to combat stress and buffer against the negative effects of cortisol, a pro-aging hormone. It also protects your body from being bombarded with stress hormones.[5] Even more good news — every sexual excitement and orgasm helps increase your DHEA. But the most exciting thing about DHEA and orgasms is this: Regular Orgasms Can Help You Live Longer!!! Researchers have shown a 50% reduction in overall mortality in those with "high orgasmic frequency." Yes, orgasms save lives![6]

Sleep — You'll see me mention sleep over and over again in this book because it is *so important* to your health. I recommend getting to bed by 10 pm every night. It is so important to your health to make your sleep cycle a non-negotiable. And, as your DHEA levels increase, you'll start to sleep better naturally, too.

Manage stress — Higher cortisol lowers DHEA. Anything you can do to calm yourself and get out of the sympathetic overdrive state (the so-called 'fight or flight response') will help balance your hormones. My favourite thing to do is download a free meditation app, or simply find a meditation exercise on YouTube and listen to it, combined with deep breathing prior to bed.

Exercise, but not too much — Overtraining, especially with cardio, can raise cortisol levels and negatively impact DHEA. So, if you've been spending hours at the gym doing cardio, you may be doing more harm than good. My suggestion would be to focus on including weight training into your exercise regime and reducing the time you spend doing cardio.

---

[5] Legros, Jean-Jacques. "Inhibitory effect of oxytocin on corticotrope function in humans: are vasopressin and oxytocin ying–yang neurohormones?." *Psychoneuroendocrinology* 26.7 (2001): 649-655.

[6] Smith, George Davey, Stephen Frankel, and John Yarnell. "Sex and death: are they related? Findings from the Caerphilly cohort study." *Bmj* 315.7123 (1997): 1641-1644.

You may also try the following supplements to naturally increase DHEA:

- DHEA itself is a restricted substance in Canada, but is readily available over the counter in the United States. Due to the potential negative consequences and risk of taking this hormone, you should speak with a licensed health care provider and test to see if a true deficiency exists.
- Stress product: One of my favourite ways to modulate the stress response and help your body to become more resilient to stress is to use the product Adrenotone™ by Designs for Health. Adrenotone™ is a comprehensive blend of nutrients and botanical compounds designed to support healthy adrenal function.

CHAPTER FOUR

The Thyroid

Y OUR ADRENAL HORMONES ARE COMPLETELY INTERTWINED WITH THE HORMONES PRODUCED BY YOUR THYROID GLAND. They cannot be viewed in isolation, as one impacts the other profoundly. As you read this chapter, you'll notice that many of the symptoms you'll feel from an imbalance in adrenal hormones are the same as the symptoms of thyroid hormone imbalance.

Remember that all of these glands play a part in hypothalamic-pituitary-adrenal dysfunction. So, although we're addressing different hormones in separate chapters, they're all intimately interlinked. Changes in adrenal hormones will affect your thyroid hormones, and vice versa. Try to keep this in mind as you continue to read this book.

The Thyroid Gland

The thyroid sits in the front of your neck and is butterfly-shaped.

This gland plays a critical role in metabolism, mood, hormones, and cognition. The thyroid sets your body's thermostat, daily energy expenditure, growth, fertility, metabolism, skin health, and reproductive functions. It determines how easily you can lose weight, whether or not you can achieve and maintain a healthy pregnancy and lactate, as well as your mood and capability to experience joy vs. anxiety and depression. It also affects your brain's ability to remember and focus, and much more.

Thyroid Hormones, T3 and T4

The thyroid impacts all the functions listed above through the production of two important hormones: triiodothyronine (T3) and thyroxine (T4). T4 is produced in greater amounts, but T3 is the active form, made from the conversion of T4 to T3 throughout the body, especially in the liver and gut.

In order for your thyroid to produce appropriate levels of hormone, it needs a signal from the pituitary, located in the brain. The pituitary produces thyroid stimulating hormone (TSH) to tell the thyroid it's time to get moving. Once your thyroid receives the signal and produces sufficient hormones, those hormones signal the pituitary, telling it to put the brakes on creating TSH. As you can imagine, if at any point in this feedback loop anything becomes disrupted, a whole host of symptoms will ensue.

What Affects the Thyroid?

Now that you know how the thyroid gland works, let's discuss how your lifestyle and environment can affect its function. Just like with the adrenal glands, your lifestyle can have a huge impact on how well your thyroid works. So, to learn how to balance your thyroid hormones, it's important to learn what's affecting them in the first place.

Factors that inhibit proper thyroid function include:

- Stress
- Infections
- Trauma
- Radiation
- Medications
- Fluoride (acts as an antagonist to iodine)
- Toxins
- Pesticides
- Chloride
- Bromide
- Mercury
- Cadmium
- Lead
- Autoimmune disease, including celiac disease

These factors can affect many parts of thyroid function, including how thyroid hormones are synthesized, how the thyroid receives signals from the brain to make more hormones, and more.

One of the main reasons why people experience symptoms of thyroid dysfunction is their thyroid is not properly converting the hormone T4 into T3. Instead, the thyroid converts T4 to rT3, or inactive thyroid hormone. rT3 production is increased by:

- Stress
- Trauma
- Low calorie diets
- Inflammation
- Toxins
- Infections
- Liver/kidney disease
- Certain medications

If you suspect your body may not be properly converting T4 to T3, seek out a Naturopathic Doctor or a Functional Medicine Specialist who will help you get the answers you're looking for.

Exercise and Thyroid Hormones

Your diet and nutrition plan could be affecting your thyroid hormone levels. As a practitioner, one thing I educate my clients on is the dangers of over-exercising while under-eating. There are many misconceptions that I help to dispel, such as "fat does not make you fat, sugar does," as well as "not all carbs are bad."

When you don't eat enough to fuel your workouts or you don't give your body time to recover between workouts, your hormones change and inflammation occurs in the body. This can lead to fatigue, fat storage, hormone changes, and chronic disease. This is when we start to see symptoms of adrenal fatigue, subclinical hypothyroidism, or even frank hypothyroidism. I want you to know that if you have been living this way, it isn't your fault. There is a lot of confusing and often inaccurate information out there.

Over the last couple years, I have seen the fitness industry promoting "INSANE" workouts paired with a calorie-deficit nutrition plan. While I love an intense, sweat-like-no-other workout, the issue is that doing this daily will ultimately lead to some serious health issues.

Hypothyroidism & Hashimoto's

So, what happens when your thyroid isn't working properly? Hypothyroidism is the most common thyroid disturbance in North America. It refers to a decreased thyroid function or decreased thyroid hormones. The broad category of hypothyroidism can be separated into non-autoimmune thyroid disease, which is often just called hypothyroidism, and autoimmune thyroid disease, known as Hashimoto's thyroiditis or Hashimoto's. Hashimoto's disease is by far the most common form of hypothyroidism.

In Hashimoto's thyroiditis, the body's immune system attacks the thyroid. White blood cells called lymphocytes accumulate in the thyroid. Once in the thyroid, the lymphocytes make antibodies that damage the thyroid and interfere with its ability to produce thyroid hormones.

Non-autoimmune thyroid disease is not an autoimmune condition, and may be caused by nutritional deficiencies, excess iodine, or overexposure to certain foods. Chronic or severe stress can negatively impact the pituitary and affect the signaling pathways to the thyroid.

In some cases, the body's conversion of inactive T4 to active T3 is sluggish. In other cases, the body will make sufficient hormones but the active T3 gets converted to inactive reverse T3 (rT3). This is essentially the storage form of thyroid hormone and can also lead to symptoms of hypothyroidism.

Stages of Autoimmune Thyroid Disease

In an ideal world, women would be diagnosed with Hashimoto's before their thyroid lab values became significantly impacted. The goal should be to identify the underlying immune system attacking the thyroid before hypothyroidism develops. You can think of thyroid disease as a progression, and below are the common stages you may experience.

Stage 0: Many of us have genetic predispositions to develop Hashimoto's, but what determines exactly who expresses the disease and who does not has yet to be confirmed. Scientists have identified some predisposing genes and specific triggers that may cause these genes to turn on, but the exact mechanism remains unclear.

Stage 1: This is where the immune system begins to malfunction. Instead of expressing tolerance to self, the immune system begins to mount an immune attack and release antibodies against the thyroid gland. Thyroid antibodies such as Thyroid peroxidase antibody (TPO) and Thyroglobulin antibody (TGAb) can be elevated for years before changes to other lab markers occur. At this phase, even though your TSH, T3, and T4 levels are normal, you may be beginning to experience symptoms. You likely will visit your doctor and be told that you look great on paper and even be misdiagnosed with anxiety, depression, or situational fatigue.

Stage 2: In stage 2, thyroid stimulating hormone (TSH) begins to slowly rise. Unfortunately, conventional lab reference ranges are far too wide and patients suffer with symptoms for far too long using a "let's wait and see" approach.

Stage 3: TSH continues to rise as the levels of thyroid hormone T3 and T4 fall. In other cases, TSH is slightly elevated and T4 is normal, but T3 (active thyroid hormone) falls below normal. This complexity often results in misdiagnosis, as active thyroid hormone T3 testing is rarely ordered. This is where many people are experiencing many symptoms, a diagnosis is made, and artificial thyroid medications are recommended.

Stage 4: This is an overlooked but important stage. If lifestyle factors are not addressed in individuals with Hashimoto's, the risk of developing additional autoimmune disease increases. This is a big reason why taking a pill is not the best solution. Dietary and lifestyle changes are necessary.

Why Early Diagnosis is Key

In the best-case scenario, patients can use dietary and lifestyle factors to reduce their risk of developing autoimmune conditions as much as possible. If autoimmunity does begin to occur, there are lifestyle, supplement, and dietary recommendations that can be made to reverse disease progression and address symptoms.

Many studies demonstrate that antibodies are elevated and can be detected for as much as a decade before changes to TSH can be detected by conventional laboratory tests. This is why TSH alone is an inadequate screening test, and as a medical community we must do better.

The Connection Between Gallbladder Dysfunction and Your Thyroid

More and more, we are becoming aware of the connections between organ systems. For instance, subclinical hypothyroidism, meaning you likely express symptoms but your TSH is "normal," is more common among those with bile duct stones and gallbladder dysfunction.

A study out of the Tampere University Hospital in Finland investigated the prevalence of previously undiagnosed subclinical hypothyroidism in those with gallstones patients compared to non-gallstone controls.[7] The researchers found that 5.3% of the gallstone patients had under-functioning thyroid glands, compared to only 1.4% in the control group. In women over 60 years of age, the prevalence of subclinical hypothyroidism was as high as 11.4% in the gallstone group, compared to 1.8% among those who did not.

The exact reason for this association is unknown, but there are multiple factors that may contribute to the formation and/or accumulation of gall stones in hypothyroid patients, including decreased liver cholesterol metabolism, diminished bile secretion, and reduced sphincter of Oddi relaxation.

The reason I highlight the gallbladder-thyroid connection is because if a patient is experiencing gallstones or has had their gallbladder removed, I almost always investigate their thyroid

---

[7] Laukkarinen, Johanna, Juhani Sand, and Isto Nordback. "The Underlying Mechanisms: How Hypothyroidism Affects the Formation of Common Bile Duct Stones—A Review." HPB Surgery 2012 (2012).

function. I run a comprehensive lab assessment, because we can detect subclinical hypothyroidism up to 10 years prior to seeing changes to TSH (the screening marker used in conventional medicine). It is important, in my opinion, to pick it up any changes to thyroid function as soon as possible because in my experience we can reverse disease and slow progression.

In addition, since the gallbladder stores bile, which aids in the digestion of fats, it is especially important to ensure proper gallbladder function since our hormones are derived from components of fats. Bile is also important to help absorb the fat-soluble vitamins A, E, D, and K.

If you do not have a gallbladder, you may want to consider supplementing with a digestive enzyme that contains ox bile, as well as the fat-soluble vitamins listed above. Note that ox bile is not a vegetarian product, and you must be cautious when using vitamin A in pregnancy. Also, many digestive enzymes contain HCl, which you would want to be cautious with if you have ulcers, *H. pylori,* or are on a proton pump inhibitor (PPI).

Do You Have Hypothyroidism?

At this point, you've probably wondering if some of the symptoms you experience on a regular basis could be due to hypothyroidism. Take the following questionnaire to help you determine whether you should get additional screening to see if you have decreased thyroid function.

History

- I have a family history of thyroid disease.
- I've had changes to my thyroid previously.
- A member of my family currently has or has been diagnosed with an autoimmune disease.
- I have had radiation to my head, neck, chest, and/or tonsil area.

- I grew up near a nuclear power plant.
- I have a history of miscarriage or infertility.

Signs & Symptoms

- My normal body temperature is low (less than 98.2°F when I take it).
- I am gaining weight for no clear reason, or am unable to lose weight with clean eating and exercising.
- I feel fatigued and exhausted more than normal.
- I have a slow pulse or low blood pressure.
- I have high cholesterol.
- My hair is rough, coarse, dry, or breaking.
- I am losing more hair than normal.
- My skin is rough, coarse, dry, scaly, or itchy.
- My voice has become hoarse.
- I have aches, pains, stiffness or tingling in joints, muscles, hands or feet.
- My eyebrows are thinning on the outside.
- I have low sex drive.
- I feel depressed, irritable, or moody.
- I am constipated (less than one bowel movement per day)
- My eyes feel gritty, dry, and/or light sensitive.
- My neck feels full, with pressure or is larger than usual.
- I have difficulty swallowing.
- I have puffiness and swelling around the eyes, eyelids, face, hands, or feet.
- I have irregular cycles (longer, heavier, or more frequent).

If you found yourself saying "yes" to the above symptoms, I would highly recommend you contact your primary care provider for comprehensive laboratory testing. To start, at the Wild Side we run a full thyroid panel, which includes T3, T4, TSH, thyroid antibodies, and rT3, but this testing alone does not provide the full picture.

When it comes to Hashimoto's and other thyroid conditions, there are many factors that could be influencing the function of your thyroid. Factors that contribute to proper production of thyroid hormones include nutrients like iron, iodine, tyrosine, zinc, selenium, vitamin E, B2, B3, B6, C, and D. This is why at the Wild Side, we run an organic acid test on almost every patient to evaluate the function of their cellular health and uncover nutrient deficiencies.

Other factors that prevent the proper production of thyroid hormones include stress, infection, trauma, radiation, medications, fluoride (antagonist to iodine), as well as toxins like pesticides, mercury, cadmium, and lead. To identify any of these factors we also perform a careful evaluation of your health history, listen to your story, and may recommend specific testing such as the GI-MAP. This test is a comprehensive pathogen assay that can uncover hidden stressors, infections, and evaluate the function of your digestive system. You may be wondering…why is this important? Hippocrates famously said, *"All disease begins in the gut."* If your digestive system is not working optimally (constipation, bloating, etc.), it is virtually impossible for you to be operating at your highest level.

Improve Your Thyroid Function Naturally

What can you do to improve your thyroid function naturally? If you're worried that you might have hypothyroidism, or if your history puts you at risk and you want to reduce that risk, consider adding some of these lifestyle changes and supplements to your routine. When considering a thyroid supplement, it is best to first "test, not guess." Speak with your doctor about completing a full thyroid panel (TSH, rT3, free T3, free T4, Anti-TPO antibodies, Anti-TG antibodies) as well as assessing for nutrient deficiencies like iodine, vitamin D and iron.

Nutrients That Contribute to Proper Thyroid Function:

- Iron

- Iodine
- Tyrosine
- Zinc
- Selenium
- Vitamin E
- Vitamin B2
- Vitamin B3
- Vitamin B6
- Vitamin C
- Vitamin D

On top of keeping your thyroid gland healthy, you can also help the cells in your thyroid convert T4 to the active thyroid hormone T3.

Nutrients that increase conversion of T4 to T3:

- Selenium
- Zinc

In addition to the supplements listed above, there are changes you can make and supplements you can take to help cells throughout your body be more sensitive to thyroid hormones. This is important because the action or outcome of thyroid hormone is dependent not only upon thyroid hormone being produced, but also on binding to receptors on target cells. Just like type 2 diabetes occurs when your cells aren't sensitive to insulin anymore, your cells need to be sensitive to thyroid hormones to function properly.

Nutrients that improve cellular sensitivity to thyroid hormones:

- Vitamin A
- Exercise
- Zinc

CHAPTER FIVE

Sex Hormones

AS WOMEN, OUR SEX HORMONES NATURALLY FLUCTUATE MONTHLY. Our menstrual cycles are actually very complex and must be orchestrated precisely so we can feel our best. Lifestyle factors such as eating inflammatory foods or not getting enough sleep can have profound impacts hormonally. I know! It's kind of a bummer, but luckily there are simple strategies you can implement to begin getting your hormones back on track.

Sex Hormones in Women

Estrogen and progesterone are the main female sex hormones. Estrogen is present in both men and women. When we have appropriate amounts of estrogen in our bodies, especially in relation to other hormones like cortisol, insulin, and progesterone, all is well. Estrogen is thought of as the "feminine" hormone and gives women their female characteristics like breast tissue and hips.

Estrogen is important in the first half of the menstrual cycle for the growth and development of the uterine lining, but too much estrogen can also stimulate pathological growth. In fact, long-term effects of estrogen overload include an increased risk of breast, uterine, and endometrial cancers, as well as atypical pap smears.

When estrogen and progesterone are out of balance, they are rarely the only ones. In fact, your hormonal imbalance may stem from issues with your thyroid, adrenals, liver, gut, diet, and lifestyle factors.

Women also produce androgens, which most people think of as the male sex hormones. Hormones that fall into this category are testosterone, DHEA, and androsterone. Although we do usually associate these hormones with men, they're still very important to women's health. Typically, women have lower testosterone than men, but levels can be elevated in conditions such as polycystic ovary syndrome (PCOS).

Back in Chapter 3, we discussed the importance of DHEA. DHEA is a precursor to both estrogen and testosterone, and it has an extensive benefit list. It is known to support the immune system, sleep, muscle growth, fat loss, and can counteract the negative effects of cortisol. It also is known for having anti-aging effects, and increasing libido and enhancing motivation.

Because we are a whole people and every part of us is connected, I rarely, if ever, only address female sex hormones when patients come see me looking to restore balance.

Why Sex Hormone Balance is Important

Like any of the other hormones in your body, it's incredibly important to support sex hormone balance. If your hormones are out of whack, you're not alone. Imbalances of the female hormones progesterone and estrogen are quite common and often difficult to correct.

Hormone imbalances can present themselves in some interesting ways. Some signs your system is out of whack are feeling tired throughout the day, difficulties concentrating or brain fog, inability to lose weight, and inexplicably feeling down.

Are you unsure whether you're experiencing an imbalance of the female sex hormones (estrogen and progesterone)? Check your symptoms against these lists of common signs of imbalance:

High Estrogen

- Weight gain
- Fibrocystic breasts
- Heavy or irregular menses
- Breast tenderness
- Irritability and frustration
- Bloating
- Water retention
- Acne
- Headache

Low Estrogen

- Hot flashes
- Night sweats
- Anxiety and depression
- Insomnia
- Osteoporosis
- Vaginal dryness
- Decrease in libido
- Incontinence
- Hair loss

- Cardiovascular disease

High Progesterone

- Irritability
- Long menstrual cycle
- Fatigue
- Headache
- Breast tenderness
- Emotional changes

Low Progesterone

- Anxiety
- Irritability
- Menstrual cramps
- Irregular or heavy cycle
- Fibrocystic breasts
- Insomnia

If you can identify with some or many of the above symptoms, you may be experiencing hormone imbalances. The key to healthy hormones is to support the whole body, with a special focus on ovaries, adrenals, and thyroid. A multi-system approach incorporating diet, lifestyle, lab testing, physical exams, stress management, and sleep is ideal.

Your ovaries, thyroid, and adrenals all need to be functioning optimally together to restore hormone balance. These glands work together like a three-legged stool. If one leg is weak or missing, the stool is not strong, and the whole system risks collapse.

If you have been experiencing symptoms of hormone imbalance – fatigue, acne, weight changes, PMS, anxiety or depression, then you'll likely benefit from supporting all three legs of the stool. Follow the suggestions in Chapters 3, 4, and 5 of this book and you'll be on your way to balancing your hormones and improving your overall health.

Testing for Sex Hormone Imbalance

Are your sex hormones to blame for the symptoms you're experiencing? The key to helping you feel better is identifying where the imbalances are occurring! This often requires a detailed history as well as lab testing to determine which organs are in need of support. In addition, comprehensive lab testing allows for the best individualized plan to be developed for you.

Testing that may be recommended includes:

- Dutch Test — dried urine test
- Estradiol, FSH, LH (Best tested on Day 3 of your menstrual cycle.) — blood test
- Progesterone (Best tested on Day 19-22 of your menstrual cycle.) — blood test
- Thyroid panel: TSH, Free T4, Free T3, Reverse T3, Anti-TPO, Anti-thyroglobulin — blood test
- Free Testosterone — blood test
- Sex Hormone Binding Globulin — blood test

Additional testing may be necessary based on your individual needs. For instance, the GI Map test may be necessary to evaluate if your estrogen is being recycled by measuring betaglucoxoidation levels.

How Sex Hormones Affect Your Weight

Did you notice that weight gain was listed as one of the potential symptoms of sex hormone imbalance? Many women struggle to lose weight because their sex hormones are out of balance. This will be particularly true for you if you are estrogen dominant.

If you are someone who has been eating clean and exercising, but you cannot seem to lose the weight, or you are someone who loses five then gains back eight, you may be dealing with estrogen dominance. When hormones are out of whack, losing weight is very challenging, to the point of being almost impossible and often disappointing.

Having a lot of estrogen in your body tends to make your cells less sensitive to insulin. When your cells don't respond to insulin like they should, they don't take up sugars that your body uses for energy from your blood. So, what does your body do with all of those unused sugars? It starts to store them as fat. So, even if you're eating well and exercising, you can still gain weight (and a lot of it) if you're estrogen dominant.

Risk Factors for Developing Estrogen Dominance

Age — At some point in their mid-thirties, women begin to produce less estrogen as their ovarian reserves decrease. But, estrogen levels don't provide a clear picture on their own. Instead, you need to look at your estrogen levels relative to the amount of progesterone you have in your body. Estrogen and progesterone oppose one another and work harmoniously throughout our cycles. If progesterone is low, that is going to show up as a relative estrogen dominance in the body and produce the symptoms of estrogen dominance.

Stress — Stress management, sleep, and mindset are critical, but their value is often underappreciated. Remember that when you are in a constant state of stress, at least initially, your cortisol levels will be high. Cortisol is produced at the expense of progesterone and other important sex hormones like DHEA. Supplementing with progesterone may fix the issue temporarily, but if the root cause is a cortisol issue, then this should be addressed.

Impaired Liver Function — Back in Chapter 2 we learned that the liver is where hormones and toxins are conjugated and prepared for excretion. Under normal circumstances, the liver performs well and does not require extra support. But if your liver is not performing up to bar hormone imbalances may result. Go back and read through Chapter 2 to learn how you can help enhance your liver's natural ability to remove excess sex hormones.

Poor Gut Health — There is new fascinating research emerging that suggests the foods we eat directly change and influence our microbiome. The microbiome is the aggregate of microbes that live in your gut. We now know your microbiome plays a major role in your risk of diseases such as obesity, cancer, and diabetes.[8] The more of the hormone-damaging foods you consume, the more you are promoting the growth of the wrong bacteria in your gut, a double whammy. These "wrong bacteria" impact estrogen by causing estrogen to be recycled. We can measure estrogen recycling by testing beta-glucuronidase with the GI Map test.

Exposure to Environmental Estrogens — Chemicals and compounds resembling natural estrogens can overburden our bodies' abilities to detox and eliminate estrogens. I'm not just talking about the Pill (more on that soon) — your plastics, water, foods (particularly meat and alcohol), canned foods, personal care products, and cleaning supplies may all contain chemicals that resemble estrogen or that raise estrogen levels in the body.

Constipation — Our hormones, as well as toxins, are excreted from our bodies through our bowels. If you are not having at least one large bowel movement a day, chances are your hormones are being reabsorbed.

How to Use Your Menstrual Cycle to Lose Fat

Our menstrual cycle and fluctuations in hormone levels absolutely affect our metabolism, how our bodies utilize nutrients, as well as our

---

[8] Parazzini, F. et al. "Diet and endometriosis risk: a literature review." *Reproductive Biomedicine Online* 26, no. 4 (2013): 323-336.

physical performance. In order to maximize our efforts, we must strategically align our workouts and nutrition regimes with the ebb and flow in our hormones.

The menstrual cycle causes large shifts in female hormones which can result in changes to:

- Mood
- Energy
- Sex drive
- Hunger
- Strength
- Cravings and appetite
- How our bodies use fuel
- Risk of injury

In order to optimize your body composition, you should be aware of these changes and know how to customize your program to match your hormone changes when needed. This is what I am going to show you how to do later in this book, so you can work out smarter not harder and thus reach your goals faster with less effort!

The Follicular Phase

The follicular phase is the first two weeks of your cycle, or up until ovulation occurs. This is the perfect time to schedule your more intense training and workouts that incorporate lifting heavy weights. Interestingly, research show that your pain tolerance, strength, and endurance are higher during this time.[9] Because you are able to step up the intensity of your exercise during this time, it warrants priority given to refeed days or additional carbohydrate consumption.

To further support additional carb intake, evidence shows women have improved insulin sensitivity during this time of their cycles,

---

[9] Riley III, Joseph L., et al. "A meta-analytic review of pain perception across the menstrual cycle." *Pain* 81.3 (1999): 225-235.

allowing you to utilize carbs more within your muscles. Remember insulin works as a carrier, shunting nutrients and digested carbs (predominantly in the form of blood sugar) into your muscles. Thus, prioritizing healthy carbs during this time is key to optimize the metabolic state and maximize the benefits of those additional carbs. Make sure you're eating your highest carb meal 1-2 hours after your workout to really get the best results. Post workout meal is ½ plate of veggies, 4-6 oz protein, and a palm-size portion of a gluten-free carb source such as sweet potatoes, rice, oats, and so on.

The Luteal Phase

The luteal phase occurs from the time of ovulation to the start of your next cycle. This is where you will likely notice the biggest impact on your performance and energy. You may need to reduce the weights a bit or take additional active recovery days.

Some big physiological changes are occurring. Firstly, your basal body temperature increases, and thermogenesis increases along with it. Personally, I notice my body will burn an additional 5-10% more calories during the luteal phase, and this is fairly typical. This unfortunately does not warrant increased food intake, specifically for women looking to lose fat. Note that women who are no longer cycling will need to adjust diet and lifestyle because they no longer have this increase.

Secondly, due to the nature of the hormones in this phase, you may notice water retention and bloating. DO NOT GET ON THE SCALE! The scale, in my opinion, is actually the worst tool to assess progress because there are too many variables that affect total weight. You will absolutely be heavier this week, but it means nothing — it is just water weight, and it will pass!

Thirdly, research shows reduced insulin sensitivity and carbohydrate tolerance during this time. This is a great week to experiment with a lower carbohydrate or ketogenic-type plan. Cravings may be higher at this time, but let's be real — it's not ideal to dabble in just one bite of chocolate during the time when your hormones are making you crave it the most.

Lastly, in addition to hormone changes, serotonin (a neurotransmitter in the brain controlling mood) may drop. This may be the culprit if you experience changes to mood, behaviour, and/or irritability. You may notice increase cravings for carbs because these will elevate serotonin in the short term. Recognize this as a normal part of your physiology and try to prevent giving in to your cravings as much as possible. To reduce cravings, increase your intake of water, protein, and leafy greens. You can also eat more foods that contain tryptophan, which is a precursor to serotonin, or consider supplementation.

The Pill — the Bad, and the Ugly

If you think your contraception is free from side effects other than preventing pregnancy, think again. Hormonal contraceptives are known to affect every aspect of your body. The Pill can also cause an array of symptoms like anxiety, depression, low libido, weight gain, and digestive issues.

In addition, many women experience negative symptoms of the Pill even after they stop taking it. These symptoms range from heavy, painful periods to absent periods and hair loss, all symptoms they may or may not have had prior to starting the Pill. In fact, all of the following symptoms are associated with *coming off* of the birth control Pill:

- Post-Pill amenorrhea (loss of menstruation after taking the pill)
- Heavy menstruation
- Painful periods
- Short menstrual cycles (<24 days)
- Infertility
- Hypothyroidism

- Hair loss
- Breast tenderness
- Acne
- Adrenal dysfunction
- Pain syndromes like migraines and headache
- Weight gain or difficulty losing weight
- Mood disorders such as anxiety, depression
- Mood swings
- Digestive upset, gas, or bloating
- Inflammation and other immune imbalances

The good news is your body can reverse these symptoms and can heal! The first step is to start optimizing your liver function. Hormonal contraceptives contain synthetic hormones that must be processed by your liver in order for your body to remove them from your system. This is the main mechanism of detoxification that your body uses to eliminate hormones that are no longer needed.

Supporting detoxification and elimination is one of the key components of restoring hormone balance. We will briefly review ways to support detox here but for a deeper understanding, refer back to Chapter 2.

Why Support Your Liver & Bowels?

Your liver is responsible for getting hormones ready to be moved out by the gut, which means it must be working at its best if you want to balance your hormones. High levels of synthetic estrogen require additional work by the liver to process them so your body can eliminate them. It's no secret the Pill and other synthetic hormones take a toll on this very important organ.

Once the liver has done its job, the excess hormones must be eliminated through the bowels. This is why I am adamant that my clients must have a bowel movement every day. If you're not having at least one bowel movement a day, then you need to find out why. Many people report constipation relief by increasing their daily fibre intake (eating more fruits and vegetables), consuming more water, or taking magnesium bisglycinate nightly. Others need support through the use of a prokinetic like ginger, 5HTP and B6.

Eating for Estrogen Detox

Since the liver is a key player in estrogen detox, I recommend eating foods that provide nutrients to support liver function. These foods include:

- Beets
- Burdock root
- Dandelion root tea
- Garlic
- Complete proteins
- Cruciferous vegetables

Eating a whole-food diet with a minimum of 3-6 cups of vegetables and lean proteins will provide your liver with essential nutrients it needs to support your natural detox pathways. Protein is critical for detox. If you are not getting enough in your diet, add a protein amino acid supplement.

Next, is it important to eat organic when possible. Pesticides and herbicides used on non-organic foods must be processed by the liver, which puts it under additional stress. In addition, make sure you choose pasture-raised meats, as well as free-range eggs. These foods are also less likely to contain chemicals that put unnecessary stress on your liver.

Also ensure you are consuming a diet with adequate amounts of healthy fats such as avocado, cold-pressed olive oil, coconut oil, macadamia nut oil, olives, and so on. These healthy fats have been shown to support liver health.[10]

Finally, if you're not already getting half your body weight in ounces of fluid daily, definitely start there. A good rule is to up your intake of water by about 20 extra ounces per day during a detox.

All of the above recommendations will ensure you keep your blood sugar balanced and you supply your body with the fuel it needs to create hormones, and to remove excess hormones from your body.

Supplements to Consider for Detox

At the Wild Side Wellness, we use professional-grade detoxification support for 14-28 days to support the body in optimizing hormone balance and improving health quickly. This phase is foundational, and I've seen women who struggle with hormonal symptoms even years after going off of the Pill benefit from starting with a detox. Depending on your unique symptoms you may benefit from liver support that stimulates both phase 1 and 2 detoxification pathways or you may be recommended nutraceuticals that promote estrogen balance like DIM or calcium-D-glucarate. Keep in mind hormones like estrogen must be eliminated through the bowels, so an optimal gut microbiome and sufficient bowel movements are key.

How to Support Your Liver on the Pill

If you're currently on the Pill and plan to continue with it, the same principles as above will apply. Eat plenty of cruciferous vegetables, including cauliflower, broccoli, and kale. In addition, focus on consuming 4-6 oz of lean protein and a few tablespoons of healthy

---

[10] Gupta, Vikas, et al. "Oily fish, coffee and walnuts: Dietary treatment for nonalcoholic fatty liver disease." *World Journal of Gastroenterology: WJG* 21.37 (2015): 10621.

fats at every meal. You too can benefit from a 14-day detox. For the women who chose to continue with the Pill, I recommend supporting your liver with a detox program every 3-6 months and monitoring for nutrient deficiencies. A B vitamin complex, magnesium and zinc are especially important at this time.

Treating PCOS Naturally

PCOS is an acronym for Polycystic Ovarian Syndrome or Polycystic Ovary Syndrome. It is the most common endocrine disorder that affects women of reproductive age in North America.[11] As many as 1 in 10 women suffer from PCOS — that is at least 5 million women in US alone! Hashimoto's is even more common, but we think of it as more of an autoimmune condition.

PCOS is considered triad of amenorrhea (lack of a menstrual cycle over a number of cycles without pregnancy or menopause), obesity, and hirsutism (male pattern hair growth, unwanted facial hair).[12] Initially, PCOS was thought to be a hormonal or a sex hormone endocrine problem, but now we know it is really much more of a metabolic condition. The root of the problem is not necessarily progesterone, estrogen, or testosterone, but rather insulin resistance.

At the cellular level in PCOS there is insulin resistance, which results is hyperinsulinemia (high insulin in the blood). Your pancreas is producing the insulin, but the cellular uptake is not happening because of the cellular resistance. As a result, you have excess circulating insulin (hyperinsulinemia).

Hyperinsulinemia is an issue as it leads to stimulation of the ovaries and hyperandrogenism (remember, testosterone is an

---

[11] Williams, Tracy, Rami Mortada, and Samuel Porter. "Diagnosis and Treatment Of Polycystic Ovary Syndrome". *Aafp.org*. N.p., 2017. Web. 26 May 2017.
[12] Sirmans, Susan M., and Kristen A. Pate. "Epidemiology, diagnosis, and management of polycystic ovary syndrome." *Clinical epidemiology* 6 (2014): 1.

androgen) and also decreased synthesis of sex hormone binding globulin (SHBG).[10] SHBG is a protein in serum that binds to a number of different hormones (sex hormones and active thyroid hormone). When hormones are bound to SHBG, they are functionally ineffective.

But, what does high insulin have to do with your sex hormones?

High levels of circulating insulin stimulate the ovaries to secrete testosterone and stop the liver from producing SHBG. Recall that SHBG binds hormones and renders them inactive. Higher testosterone production and lower SHBG results in high circulating androgen levels, including testosterone.

This accounts for cystic acne (mostly along the jawline, cheeks, chin), facial hair, and male pattern hair loss that many women with PCOS experience. These "cosmetic" symptoms are what cause the most tremendous social impact, lack of confidence, and anxiety/depression in women with PCOS.

Signs & Symptoms of PCOS

The following symptoms are common in women who have PCOS:

- Irregular periods, no periods, or not ovulating with each cycle
- Multiple follicles developing at the same time on ovaries seen on ultrasound (known as a "string of pearls")
- Infertility
- Signs of elevated androgens (acne, hirsutism, male pattern baldness)
- Weight gain or inability to lose weight
- Acanthosis nigricans – discolouration or darkening around the skin folds (on the neck, under fat folds)
- Depression, anxiety, and eating disorders, especially binge eating (likely to do with the blood sugar dysregulation)

Diagnosis of exclusion — determined by the Rotterdam Criteria – 2 out of the 3 following are required to make a diagnosis of PCOS:[13]

- Irregular or no menstrual cycle
- Observation of signs of hyperandrogenism (acne, hirsutism, male pattern baldness) OR laboratory indications
- Polycystic ovaries (by ultrasound)

It is important to note that while lab tests can be used to confirm PCOS (LH, FSH, and testosterone), but *normal labs do not exclude the condition*. This is because lab testing can be very variable based on when in the month the labs were completed, your current weight and many other factors.

Treatment for PCOS

Proper treatment of PCOS can bring about many benefits, including:

- Improvement symptoms of excess androgens (hirsutism, acne, male pattern hair loss)
- Prevention of endometrial cancer (your risk of endometrial cancer increases when you are chronically not ovulating)
- Management of the metabolic abnormalities to reduce risk of type 2 diabetes and cardiovascular disease
- Improvement of fertility and pregnancy outcomes

So how is PCOS treated? Conventional treatment of PCOS usually involves the use of one or more of the following therapies:

Oral Contraceptives — The birth control pill is commonly recommended to reduce male hormone levels and regulate a women

---

[13] McLuskie, Isabel, and Aisha Newth. "New Diagnosis of Polycystic Ovary Syndrome". *BMJ* (2017): i6456. Web.

cycle. There are risks of using oral contraceptive pills (OCP), which should be discussed with your doctor. While OCP reduces male sex hormones, it has been shown to negatively affect insulin sensitivity, as well as lipid and carbohydrate metabolism. Worsening the underlying cause of PCOS, in my opinion, may not be the best approach.

Spironolactone — This drug acts as an anti-androgen and helps to lower male hormones and improve symptoms of androgen excess (hirsutism, acne, male pattern hair loss)

Metformin — This drug is typically used for diabetics. It has anti-inflammatory effects, regulates insulin levels, supports a pregnancy, and may restore menstrual cycles in women with PCOS.

Okay, so we know what PCOS & insulin sensitivity is, and we know what the conventional treatments are. Now, what are some natural prescriptions used to treat PCOS?

1. Lose Weight

This might be a no-brainer, but those who have a lower body fat percentage see marked improvements in insulin sensitivity over those who are overweight. One of the many challenges with losing weight with PCOS is sugar cravings. Cravings are mostly due to the dysregulation of blood glucose. I have meal plans to help you curb sugar cravings that you may find helpful; you can find them on my website at breannekallonen.com/shop. If you are struggling with cravings, get help. I have been there, and you shouldn't have to use superhuman willpower.

Research shows that an average loss of 13.9 lbs. leads to decreased fasting insulin and testosterone levels. In this same study 92% (12/13) of the PCOS women resumed ovulation and 85% (11/13) became pregnant.[14]

---

[14] McLuskie, Isabel, and Aisha Newth. "New Diagnosis Of Polycystic Ovary Syndrome". *BMJ* (2017): i6456. Web.

2. Weight Train

Multiple studies have found increases in insulin sensitivity when weight training is applied to a regular workout routine.[15,16,17] Weight training also increases your muscle mass, further benefiting your metabolism and hormone levels.

3. Build Muscle

This goes hand in hand with weight training, but one of the reasons that weight training stimulates an increase in insulin sensitivity is that lifting weights builds muscle. With more muscle, you will have more space to store carbs in the form of glycogen, and your metabolism will be faster.

4. Tailor Your Nutrition

If you are an individual starting a diet with an extremely high amount of body fat, you may want to consider a higher fat, lower carb approach to dieting. In fact, many studies are supporting the fact that ketogenic dieting (i.e. high fat, moderate protein, very low carb dieting) leads to significant improvements in insulin sensitivity.[18,19]

---

[15] Ahmadizad, Sajad, et al. "Effects of short-term nonperiodized, linear periodized and daily undulating periodized resistance training on plasma adiponectin, leptin and insulin resistance." *Clinical biochemistry* 47.6 (2014): 417-422.

[16] Holten, Mads K., et al. "Strength training increases insulin-mediated glucose uptake, GLUT4 content, and insulin signaling in skeletal muscle in patients with type 2 diabetes." *Diabetes* 53.2 (2004): 294-305.

[17] Ishii, Tomofusa, et al. "Resistance training improves insulin sensitivity in NIDDM subjects without altering maximal oxygen uptake." *Diabetes care* 21.8 (1998): 1353-1355.

[18] Boden, Guenther, et al. "Effect of a low-carbohydrate diet on appetite, blood glucose levels, and insulin resistance in obese patients with type 2 diabetes." *Annals of internal medicine* 142.6 (2005): 403-411.

[19] Sharman, Matthew J., et al. "A ketogenic diet favorably affects serum biomarkers for cardiovascular disease in normal-weight men." *The Journal*

To start, I tell clients to download a free macro tracker (like MyFitnessPal) and aim for less than 50 grams of net carbs per day (net carbs = total carbs - fibre).

Another option that I more often recommend is carb cycling combined with intermittent fasting. In my opinion, carb-cycling would be a long-term option, where are a ketogenic diet plan may be used initially to improve insulin sensitivity. This leads to better cortisol cycles for women than a restrictive carbohydrate diet like the ketogenic diet. That being said, carbohydrates should come from quality sources like root vegetables, sweet potatoes, squash, quinoa, legumes, vegetables, and so on. We'll discuss carb cycling and intermittent fasting in greater detail later in the book.

5. Assess Your Overall Nutrient Status

It is important to consider the entire body when treating PCOS. Addressing any nutrient deficiencies will help to improve health outcomes. I utilize organic acid testing in my practice to identify deficiencies

One deficiency I pay close attention to is magnesium. Magnesium deficiency is incredibly common — in 2009, the World Health Organization estimated that 70% of Americans are deficient in magnesium.[20] In fact, the issue of magnesium deficiency is so widespread that the WHO put out an article in 2009 looking at supplementing drinking water with calcium and magnesium. Also make sure you're not deficient in other important minerals like iron and iodine. Your diet (including supplements) should also provide your body with ample vitamins (especially B vitamins and vitamin D) and antioxidants.

In addition, vitamin D is essential for reducing insulin resistance, so if you're not getting in enough vitamin D, talk to your doctor about supplementation. Often it is recommended that blood levels be maintained between 50 and 80 for optimal health.

---

of nutrition 132.7 (2002): 1879-1885.

[20] "Calcium And Magnesium In Drinking Water: Public Health Significance". *World Health Organization*. N.p., 2009. Web. 26 May 2017.

6. Supplement Smartly

Here are a few supplements that you might consider adding to your routine to help combat PCOS:

Green Tea Extract — For some time, green tea has been known to have significant effects on improving overall health, as well as being a great supplement for burning fat. The epigallocatechin gallate (EGCG) content in green tea is what seems to be the active substance that can help the body lose fat and improve insulin sensitivity. In one study, supplementation with green tea extract compared to placebo found that the group that supplemented with the polyphenols of green tea improved insulin sensitivity by 13% when a blood glucose tolerance test was administered.[21]

D-Chiro-Inositol — Oral administration of D-chiro-inositol improves insulin sensitivity, balances blood sugar, and reduces testosterone. One study also showed that PCOS women had improved ovulation, decreased androgen levels, blood pressure and triglycerides while supplementing with D-chiro-inositol.[22] By stabilizing insulin and blood sugar, you can become more in control of your food craving and appetite. But, let's be clear: in no way will taking D-chiro-inositol make up for a high carbohydrate/high sugar diet.

A dietary source of inositol is legumes. Legumes have been associated with weight loss, improved blood sugar and reduced risk of heart disease. Examples of legumes are chickpeas (garbanzo beans), kidney beans, and non-GMO soy.

---

[21] Venables, Michelle C., et al. "Green tea extract ingestion, fat oxidation, and glucose tolerance in healthy humans." *The American journal of clinical nutrition* 87.3 (2008): 778-784.

[22] Pizzo, Alfonsa, Antonio Simone Laganà, and Luisa Barbaro. "Comparison between effects of myo-inositol and D-chiro-inositol on ovarian function and metabolic factors in women with PCOS." *Gynecological Endocrinology* 30.3 (2014): 205-208.

Chromium Picolinate — Chromium enhances insulin activity and thus plays a role in maintaining proper carbohydrate and lipid metabolism in our bodies. It has been used as a supplement to help reduce body weight and alter body composition. Evidence suggests that chromium picolinate increases lean body mass and basal metabolic rate, and decreases body fat percentage.[23] *Note: a common side effect of chromium supplementation is headaches.*

L-Carnitine — A 2014 study in PCOS women struggling to conceive looked at the effectiveness of L-carnitine on pregnancy rates.[24] Results showed that the combination of L-carnitine and clomiphene significantly improved ovulation when compared to placebo and clomiphene alone. In addition, miscarriage rates were lower in the group taking L-carnitine. Lastly, it was noted the L-carnitine group had decreases in total cholesterol, triglycerides, and LDL ("bad cholesterol"), while HDL ("good cholesterol") increased.

Cinnamon — Not only is cinnamon one of my favourite spices, but it also improves insulin resistance. A small 2014 study looked at cycle regularity and compared cinnamon versus a placebo. The group that received cinnamon had significantly more regular cycles.[25] I often add cinnamon to baked apples, smoothies, oatmeal, and coffee/tea.

7. Reduce Stress

Remember that stress increases cortisol levels in the body. Cortisol

---

[23] Pittler, M. H., C. Stevinson, and E. Ernst. "Chromium picolinate for reducing body weight: meta-analysis of randomized trials." *International journal of obesity* 27.4 (2003): 522-529.

[24] Ismail, Alaa M., et al. "Adding l-carnitine to clomiphene resistant PCOS women improves the quality of ovulation and the pregnancy rate. A randomized clinical trial." *European Journal of Obstetrics & Gynecology and Reproductive Biology* 180 (2014): 148-152.

[25] Kort, Daniel H., and Roger A. Lobo. "Preliminary evidence that cinnamon improves menstrual cyclicity in women with polycystic ovary syndrome: a randomized controlled trial." *American journal of obstetrics and gynecology* 211.5 (2014): 487-e1.

is a major synchronizing hormone for the entire hormone axis. It influences our circadian rhythm, pancreatic function, detoxification functions, inflammatory response, and insulin levels. Elevated cortisol leads to higher liberation of blood sugar, and thus higher insulin levels. Chronic stress can lead to hyperinsulinemia and insulin resistance.[26]

Lifestyle changes that can improve cortisol function are meditation, mindfulness, yoga, practicing good sleep hygiene, reducing over-exercising, carbohydrate cycling, as well as reducing stimulant intake (coffee, tea). Consider the addition of adaptogenic herbs such as Rhodiola, Ashwagandha, Schisandra, Ginseng, and Maitake mushroom, which are beneficial for adrenal support. *Note:* Maitake mushroom is not only an adaptogen, but has been shown to support women with PCOS by regulating blood sugar and insulin while inducing ovulation.[27]

8. Heal Your Gut

New evidence is emerging that there is a tremendous connection between gut health and obesity. What you have going on in your gut has a huge impact on what you are craving. (More *Candida*, for instance, makes you crave more sugar and carbs.) Our microbiome (gut bacteria) also can cross-talk with chemicals in our brain to disrupt appetite and satiety signals. Gut dysregulation also contributes to inflammation, which may predispose you to insulin resistance, PCOS, and/or obesity.[28]

---

[26] Chandola, Tarani, Eric Brunner, and Michael Marmot. "Chronic stress at work and the metabolic syndrome: prospective study." *BMJ* 332.7540 (2006): 521-525.

[27] Chen, Jui-Tung, et al. "Maitake mushroom (*Grifola frondosa*) extract induces ovulation in patients with polycystic ovary syndrome: a possible monotherapy and a combination therapy after failure with first-line clomiphene citrate." *The Journal of Alternative and Complementary Medicine* 16.12 (2010): 1295-1299.

[28] Cani, P. D., et al. "Role of gut microflora in the development of obesity and insulin resistance following high-fat diet feeding." *Pathologie Biologie* 56.5 (2008): 305-309.

For optimal health, ensure you are having at least one bowel movement every day. Remember, hormones that are metabolized in the liver must be excreted through the bowels. Slow bowels lead to recirculation of hormones back into the bloodstream, causing hormone imbalances. To ensure a daily bowel movement, make sure you are consuming enough fibre-rich fruits and vegetables. If you are reaching your daily fibre goals but still not seeing the desired results, consider a probiotic with *Lactobacillus* and *Bifidobacterium* strains (or fermented foods), magnesium bisglycinate if needed, and/or a prokinetic supplement if needed.

9. Environmental Impact and Detoxification

In order to have healthy hormone balance, we need to be effectively detoxifying and eliminating hormone toxins from our environment (xenobiotics). And, our bodies also need to eliminate the hormone toxins that are naturally occurring in our bodies (endobiotics). If our bodies are not eliminating hormones, inflammatory molecules, signaling compounds, environmental toxins and drugs from circulation, we are at increased risk for a nasty cluster of conditions known as The Western Cluster because they are so prevalent in Western societies.

Bigger issues we are seeing in our society today are pointing to toxin overload or impaired metabolic detoxification. Symptoms of these problems include earlier puberty, fibroids, endometriosis, mood changes, PCOS, type 2 diabetes, obesity, infertility, and autoimmune diseases. In my opinion, all of these diseases and symptoms have roots in environmental exposure.

To support detoxification, we want to reduce environmental exposure (plastic, flame retardants, cosmetics, household cleaners, pesticides, etc.). You should also consume foods that support detoxification, as well as try to limit your exposure to pesticides. Check out the Environmental Working Group (EWG) to learn about the Clean 15 and Dirty Dozen, the fruits and vegetables least and most likely to be covered in pesticides, respectively. Lastly, you may need to consider a botanical or antioxidant supportive detoxification program if your body's detoxification process is suspected to be significantly impaired.

If you have PCOS, the good news is that you have many natural treatment options to help your body and your hormones get back into balance. If you're really struggling with the effects of PCOS and hormone imbalance, find a specialist who can help you bring things back to where they need to be.

Ways to Treat Acne Naturally That Actually Work

Like many of you, when I am stressed and I'm eating too much sugar or dairy, my body lets me know it is not impressed by rewarding me with acne, especially along the jawline and forehead.

Let's take a closer look at why sugar and dairy contribute to acne:

Consuming dairy is an issue when it comes to acne because it can boost androgens (male sex hormones), as well as increase insulin levels.

Here's a short list of just a few of the 60-some hormones in your average glass of milk—even the organic, raw, and bovine-growth-hormone-free milk:

- 20α-dihydropregnenolone
- progesterone (from pregnenolone)
- 5α-pregnanedione
- 5α-pregnan-3β-ol-20-one,
- 20α- and 20β-dihydroprogesterone (from progesterone)
- 5α-androstene-$3\beta17\beta$-diol
- 5α-androstanedione
- 5α-androstan-3β-ol-17-one
- androstenedione
- testosterone
- dehydroepiandrosterone sulphate acyl ester

- insulin like growth factors 1 and 2 (IGF-1 and IGF-2)
- insulin

Two large controlled trials found that cow's milk increased both the number of people who got acne and its severity. Other large randomized prospective controlled trials (the gold standard of medical research) found that people who had higher sugar intake and a high glycemic load diet (more bread, rice, cereal, pasta, sugar, and flour products of all kinds) had significantly more acne. The good news is that chocolate (dark chocolate, that is) didn't seem to cause acne.

Similarly, foods that cause a quick rise in blood sugar (sugar and starchy carbs) spike insulin and elevated insulin levels can cause acne.

Every single carbohydrate you eat will eventually get converted into glucose — the form of sugar in your blood. In order to get glucose into cells to be used as energy or stored as glycogen, insulin is required. Therefore, insulin is an absolutely vital hormone for health. However, the big problem for almost everybody is not that we don't have enough insulin in our bodies, it's that we have too much. Elevated levels of insulin or multiple spikes of insulin throughout the day will stimulate sebum production. Sebum is the oil that is responsible for blocking your skin's pores. It is produced by the sebaceous glands in your skin, and insulin stimulates them to be active. The more insulin you have, the more sebum production there will be.

This makes it inevitable that your pores will get blocked and *P. acnes* bacteria will flood into the blocked pores, they will be attacked with an inflammatory response, and the surrounding pore will swell up and go red. Here is where a vicious cycle starts, because insulin leads to the creation of IGF-1, which stimulates a massive increase in sebum, and it also enhances the ability of androgens to cause acne.

In addition to dairy and sugar, nutritional deficiencies and excesses can worsen acne. Correcting common deficiencies, including low levels of healthy omega-3 anti-inflammatory fats, low levels of antioxidants such as vitamin E, zinc, and vitamin A, and including an important anti-inflammatory omega-6 fat called evening primrose oil all may be helpful in preventing and treating unwanted pimples.

The solution to the problem for acne…is NOT the birth control pill.

1. Cut out dairy: Swap out cow's milk for almond, coconut, or cashew milk, but read the label. Many milk alternatives are filled with sugar and canola oil. Butter is also considered dairy, so choose coconut oil or ghee. Ghee is clarified grass-fed butter, this means the proteins that cause inflammation have been removed.

2. Limit sugar and processed carbohydrates: Baked goods, breads, pasta…essentially everything white needs to be removed. If you need a low-carb treat, my go to are the delicious dark chocolate Cocofibre bars. These bars are loaded with vegetable fibre and offer a host of health benefits. This natural, soluble, prebiotic dietary fibre naturally supports healthy mineral absorption, bowel pH, immune system function, and composition of intestinal microbiota.

3. Practice intermittent fasting: Consuming fewer meals means fewer spikes in insulin levels. One human study showed that intermittent fasting lowered blood sugar by 3-6% and fasting insulin by 20-31%.

4. Stress less: The stress hormone cortisol is a big cause of insulin resistance. When you are stressed, it tells your body to increase glucose in your bloodstream in order to give you the energy to fight off the threat you face. More glucose in the blood means the pancreas is signaled to produce insulin. Over time, the cells stop responding to insulin and you become insulin resistant. Download the calm app and start incorporating meditation into your daily routine. Also remember to breathe deeply throughout your day.

5. Address nutritional deficiencies: Key things to consider when dealing with acne are: omega 3 fatty acids, zinc, vitamin D, vitamin B3, and vitamin A. Lab testing for nutrient status include Organic Acid Testing and Spectracell.

6. Consume ground pumpkin seeds and flax: Pumpkin seeds are antiandrogenic and provide a dose of zinc. Flax seeds help to ensure adequate bowel movements and are phytoestrogenic meaning they help to balance estrogen levels. The fibre content of flax also helps to feed to good gut bacteria.

7. Test hormone imbalances: The Dutch Test is a simple urine test that provides a significant amount of information about your hormones and hormone metabolites over the course of a day. This test allows medical professionals to discover the underlying cause of weight gain, fatigue, mood disturbances, glucose control, infertility & miscarriage, menstrual complaints, libido and more. This insight is provided by the ability of the Dutch test to detect imbalances in androgens (Testosterone, DHT, and DHEA), estrogens (E1, E2, E3), Cortisol, Progesterone, and Melatonin. This truly gives us a complete picture of hormone production, breakdown and excretion. It is not enough to just know you are low or high in a specific hormone. We need to understand the WHY. Is there a production issue, breakdown issue or excretion issue?

8. Consider taking a probiotic: The gut and skin interact, each one affecting the other through several pathways, especially the microbiome and its metabolites. Because they can interact, they also have the ability to influence one another's health, with the gut having a greater impact on skin health. There are many skin disorders that are more common in those with gut issues and vice versa. For example, rosacea has an association with SIBO, and inflammatory bowel disease (IBD) is also associated with a higher risk of developing an inflammatory skin condition, such as psoriasis, atopic dermatitis, and rosacea. Celiac disease is also associated with skin problems such as dermatitis herpetiformis. Before recommending a probiotic, I like to do a comprehensive stool test to determine which strains would be right for you using the GI-MAP stool test.

9. Spot treat as needed: In my practice, I use products with research to support acne reduction. My favourite spot treatment is the AlumierMD Acne Balancing Serum. In addition to spot treatment, ensure you are using products that best suit your individualized skin type. Register, order and collect points with code BA357A5B at www.AlumierMD.com/join.

CHAPTER SIX

Fat Hormones

WHEN MOST PEOPLE THINK ABOUT HORMONES, THEY THINK ABOUT MANY OF THE GLANDS WE'VE ALREADY DISCUSSED AND THE HORMONES THEY SECRETE. But, did you know that your body's fat cells (adipocytes) also secrete hormones? In fact, many scientists and doctors are beginning to see fat (adipose tissue) as an endocrine organ, just like the thyroid or adrenal glands.[29]

So, if we're going to have a discussion about balancing the hormones in your body and how they affect your weight, we can't ignore these hormones. Your body's adipose tissue secretes many hormones, but for the purpose of this chapter, we're going to focus on leptin, ghrelin, and adiponectin.

---

[29] Guerre-Millo, Micheie. "Adipose tissue hormones." *Journal of endocrinological investigation* 25.10 (2002): 855-861.

Leptin and Ghrelin

If you're struggling to lose fat because you're eating too much or eating the wrong foods, it is important to understand WHY you are hungry in the first place. Are you experiencing true physiological hunger, or is your body telling you that you are tired, stressed, bored, or dehydrated? Another possibility is you have created imbalances with your hunger/satiety hormones — leptin and ghrelin.

When you eat, the fat cells in your body secrete a hormone called leptin. Increasing leptin levels reduce your desire and motivation to continue eating. Within a few hours post meal, your leptin levels drop and this drop stimulates the release of a different hormone called ghrelin. Ghrelin is secreted by your stomach and pancreas and makes you feel hungry. This sounds like a pretty awesome system, right? Well, it is...until it's not!

One reason a lot of my clients have difficulty controlling their appetite or stopping after they've eaten enough is that they're leptin resistant. Leptin resistance is a vicious cycle that you must end. Overeating (hello college/university, pregnancy, Thanksgiving, and Christmas!) causes hyperleptinemia, meaning more and more leptin is being secreted by your fat cells. Eventually leptin's signal becomes less and less effective in controlling appetite, much like how insulin becomes less and less effective in a type 2 diabetic. What has actually happened is you have eaten yourself into a chronically insatiable appetite.

Interestingly, another cause of leptin resistance is chronically low caloric intake. Women who follow very calorie restricted diets actually produce less leptin than women who eat more calories.[30] So, if you have ever been on a diet, or yo-yo dieted, you have likely messed up your fat hormone levels.

---

[30] Anderlova, K., et al. "The influence of very-low-calorie diet on serum leptin, soluble leptin receptor, adiponectin and resistin levels in obese women." *Physiological research* 55.3 (2006): 277.

If leptin is doing its job and your cells respond appropriately, the satiety signals in your brain are immediately triggered and you stop feeling hungry. But when you become more leptin resistant, you also become more ghrelin sensitive, so when hunger hits, it hits hard and fast. Think of ghrelin as that little furball critter that sneaks into your brain making you crave high carb and high-fat foods. Before I fixed my hormone imbalances, that critter even could hijack my body and drive me to the nearest pizza or donut shop. Or, at least that's what it felt like at the time.

Leptin works in direct opposition to ghrelin, which is also known as the "hunger hormone." When imbalanced, ghrelin can have you reaching for unhealthy snacks regularly. When you don't get enough sleep, your ghrelin levels will increase and you will feel hungrier all day. Talk about a recipe for disaster! You should not have to use superhuman willpower to get through a day of clean eating.

In addition to spending too much time eating, other lifestyle factors such as lack of sleep, too much stress, and eating "hyperpalatable foods" such as processed and packaged foods can contribute to these hormone imbalances.

Restoring Leptin and Ghrelin Balance

First, recognize that appetite is normal. It keeps us alive and our species reproducing. But, if there is no need for physiological hunger and you have ample stored energy (from food or fat), then there's probably something wrong if you are constantly hungry. Here is what I would recommend you do:

1. Resensitize your body to leptins signals.

- Avoid ALL fructose: this is a real trigger for leptin resistance.
- Exercise, but avoid chronic cardio: do resistance training and short HIIT
- Control stress! Remember, stress raises cortisol, which not only causes your body to hold onto fat, but also messes with

many of the other hormones in your body. My favourite way to control stress is to start my day by filling out a journal. The one I use is called the 5 Minute Journal

- Get cold: cold exposure has actually been shown to improve leptin sensitivity. Consider a 2-5-minute cold shower, or alternating between hot and cold (1 min hot, 30 seconds cold). Always end your shower on cold.
- Stay consistent with these recommendations for 4-6 weeks.

2. Avoid foods that trigger hunger

- Keep sweets and snacks out of the house.
- Put food away. Don't leave it out on the counter to look at it each time you walk by.
- Avoid high carb and high glycemic index foods. These will cause a hunger spike very shortly after a meal, especially if not combined with protein and fat.
- Try to purchase single servings of trigger foods, and only purchase what you need.
- Avoid hyper palatable foods, meaning foods with multiple very strong flavors. For example, Chicago-style popcorn the cheesy, salty, sweet is the absolute worst thing you can do for your leptin levels.

3. Track your foods to create awareness.

- Use free food trackers like MyFitnessPal. You need to know what you are putting into your body. Track every day and everything, not just when you eat clean.
- Don't go crazy on nuts/seeds. Portion control is key. You can overdo "healthy foods."
- Count your snacks and don't overdo them.
- Make your own food. Many fast foods and restaurant foods are loaded with extra calories, salt, and sugar.
- Do not under-consume calories. There is research to support restricting calories actually can cause fat gain.

Adiponectin

You may not have heard of adiponectin before because it's not a hormone that a lot of people talk about. But, this protein hormone is actually very important. It reduces inflammation and burns fat. (How awesome is that?!) Adiponectin is produced and released from our fat cells and helps us burn fat by improving insulin sensitivity. "How can I boost this hormone," you ask? By consuming adequate protein, the right types of healthy fats, and doing strength training exercise.

CHAPTER SEVEN

Brain Hormones

OUR PHYSIOLOGICAL AND PSYCHOLOGICAL STATES ARE CONNECTED AND DIRECTLY IMPACT ONE ANOTHER. It is time to stop thinking of the body as disconnected organ systems. Serotonin, dopamine and melatonin are three key players in regulating appetite, cravings, mood, motivation, sleep patterns, and memory. All three are both hormones and neurotransmitters, meaning they not only have effects on the brain, but also throughout the entire body. When any of these are out of balance weight, digestion, and emotional health will be dramatically affected. Also, genetics (COMT for example), stress, poor dietary habits, lack of sleep, toxins, bacterial dysbiosis, drugs, alcohol, and caffeine can all throw these hormones out of optimal range. Over the next couple pages, we are going to be diving deeper into the roles each of these hormones play as well as ways to support healthy levels.

Serotonin: This brain chemical is best known for its role in depression but it is also very important in appetite, cravings, memory, self-esteem, pain tolerance, sleep, digestion and body temperature. Interestingly serotonin even though it is a brain chemical, the majority of it is produced in your gut. This is why when I am looking for the root cause of cravings and mood changes I evaluate gut health and I may even recommend stool testing such as a DNA stool test called GI-MAP. One way serotonin can impact weight is because when serotonin is low, we feel depressed or down and then we naturally crave sugars or starches to stimulate the production of serotonin. Also, serotonin levels tend to be lower in the winter explaining winter weight gain and the winter "blues."

Proteins→ L-Tryptophan → 5 HTP → Serotonin → Melatonin

Serotonin production is a complex pathway that not only relies on a steady source of tryptophan, but also key nutrients. When we look at the pathway to produce serotonin, we start by digesting the proteins we eat with stomach acid, which cannot be produced without plentiful zinc (a common deficiency). Vitamin B6 is also very important to producing the starting block L-Tryptophan (an amino acid).

L-Tryptophan needs the enzyme tryptophan hydroxylase and the presence of the cofactors folate, iron, calcium and vitamin B3 in order to convert to 5-HTP (5-Hydroxytryptophan).

Once 5-HTP is created, in the presence of the cofactors B6, magnesium, zinc and vitamin C, an enzyme converts it to 5-HT (5-Hydroxytryptamine), also known as serotonin.

As you can see, supporting healthy serotonin levels is complex and involves ensuring enough tryptophan intake from the diet, as well as vitamins, minerals, and a healthy gut microbiome.

Serotonin and appetite: Serotonin not only impacts cravings particularly for sugars and starches, but also plays a role in how much food we eat in a sitting and how often we feel we need to eat. In our brains there are receptors for serotonin. Serotonin activates some neurons to curb appetite and blocks other neurons that normally act to increase appetite.

Dopamine: Dopamine is the neurotransmitter that is critical for movement, memory, pleasure, behaviour, motivation, attention, sleep, mood, and learning. Low dopamine can be seen in conditions such as depression, addiction, lack of motivation/drive, and brain fog.

Melatonin: Melatonin is a hormone naturally secreted by a tiny gland in your brain. It helps regulate your body's circadian rhythm (your sleep and wake cycle). Melatonin is also an antioxidant, which protects against molecular damage by oxygen and nitrogen-based toxic reactants.

How to Support Serotonin, Dopamine, and Melatonin

Supporting healthy serotonin, dopamine, and melatonin levels will go a long way in ensuring your mood is supported, your mind is calm, and you are going through your day with energy. These three hormones are also really important for controlling both appetite and cravings.

Habits to Increase Dopamine

1. Consume protein (meat, fish, beans, nuts). These contain phenylalanine a building block of dopamine. Coffee may also stimulate dopamine release.

2. Exercise. Daily movement needs to be a non-negotiable like brushing your teeth.

3. Sex provides a nice dose of dopamine, which increases steadily to the point of orgasm and then declines. Apparently, the dopamine pathways in the brain involved in stimulating desire for both sex and food are shut down by the hormones released immediately after we

have an orgasm. Can you imagine better news for appetite and craving control?

4. Rhodiola. A great herb for memory, fatigue, stress and depression. Research suggests Rhodiola may fight depression by stimulating serotonin and dopamine. Take 200-400mg daily in the AM

5. Chaste tree (Vitex). Chaste tree has been shown to increase both dopamine and progesterone. I use this herb often in women who experience depression in combination with PMS or irregular menstrual cycles. Take 200mg of 10:1 extract each morning before breakfast.

6. L-tyrosine & phenylalanine. Both are building blocks of dopamine. Both can be stimulating (don't take after 3pm) and L-tyrosine and should be avoided in anyone with high blood pressure.

7. Sunlight. Serotonin is dependent on light. This is why seasonal affective disorder (SAD) comes into play during the winter months.

Habits to Increase Serotonin

1. Consume complex carbohydrates and protein because they contain tryptophan, which boosts serotonin. The best sources of tryptophan include rice, chia seeds, pumpkin seeds, peanuts, cottage cheese, and meats.

2. Vitamin D: The best way to get your vitamin D is through natural sunlight. A little sunshine on bare skin is great for your mood and supporting healthy vitamin D levels.

3. Exercise: Increasing your body temperature has been shown to boost serotonin. HIIT (high intensity interval training) is also amazing for mood- and serotonin-enhancing effects.

4. Massage: Incorporate a massage 1-2 times month as part of your

self-care routine.

5. 5-HTP: Before tryptophan can be converted to serotonin it must first become 5-hydroxytryptophan, or 5-HTP for short. Since 5-HTP is that much closer to serotonin, it can be an effective treatment option for depression, insomnia, and fibromyalgia. Consider taking 50-400 mg daily in divided doses.

6. Vitamin B6: B6 is an important cofactor that supports the conversion of 5-HTP to serotonin. Take 50-100 mg before bed.

7. Rhodiola: In addition to supporting natural dopamine production and secretion, Rhodiola can also help your body naturally increase serotonin levels. Take 200-400 mg daily in the AM

8. Inositol: Amazing for blood sugar management to prevent cravings, regulate insulin control and helps to alleviate anxiety and depression. Inositol powder can easily be added to smoothies or water. Take 4-12 g/day.

9. St John's Wort: Research supports the use of St John's Wort as an effective way to reduce symptoms of mild to moderate depression. It appears St John's Wort works by preventing the breakdown of serotonin in the brain. Caution should be taken when combining 5-HTP, SSRIs and St John's Wort. A daily dosage supported by research is 500-1800 mg away from food.[31]

Habits to Increase Melatonin

1. Just like you can increase serotonin with tryptophan-containing foods, you can also increase melatonin. Consume foods such as chia seeds, pumpkin seeds, walnuts, and as 100% tart cherry juice before bed.

---

[31] Lawvere, Silvana, and Martin C. Mahoney. "St. John's wort." *Am Fam Physician* 72.11 (2005): 2249-2254.

2. Change your environment. Turn off blue-emitting lights, lower the temperature, and only preform calming activities before bed. Your eyes and body need to sense calmness and darkness to signal to the brain to produce melatonin. Purchase blue-blocking glasses from Amazon, turn off electronics, and get blackout blinds to ensure proper sleep.

3. Melatonin: after changing your lifestyle to promote healthy sleep hygiene and consuming foods that contain tryptophan, consider supplementing with melatonin (1-10 mg). Note that melatonin is best absorbed when it is in the liposomal form. If you feel drowsy or foggy in the morning, try taking your melatonin earlier or lowering the dose. A common sleep support I use in my practice is called Insomnitol by Designs for Health.

Growth Hormone

Growth hormone (GH), also called somatotropin or human growth hormone, is (as the name suggests) a hormone that helps stimulate growth in animals. As we age, GH will decline and is associated with low testosterone, brittle bones, and faster aging. On the other hand, having adequate GH levels tends to be associated with vitality, more energy, more muscle, and better sex drive. Women should not worry about getting "big and bulky." In fact, having more lean muscle means you will burn more calories even at rest!

GH is secreted by the anterior lobe of the pituitary gland and stimulates the growth of essentially all tissues of the body. Once secreted, GH remains active in the bloodstream for a few minutes, then the liver converts it into growth factors, the most crucial being insulin-like growth factor (IGF-1). IGF-1 is known to have positive growth-promoting properties on every cell in the body. Because GH impacts so many cells, it plays a role in muscle growth, healing, fat loss, cardiovascular health, sleep, hair growth, libido, energy production, mood, and cognitive function.

The majority of GH is released during sleep, as well as during physical exercise. Here is why sleeping in complete darkness and avoiding artificial lights prior to bed is so important. When our eyes sense complete darkness, melatonin is released from the pineal gland. One of the results of increased melatonin release is a slight reduction in body temperature. Your body's thermostat is tightly regulated, so this slight drop results in an increase in GH. If you sleep with the lights on or in too warm of a room, your natural cool-down process will not take place. That increases the risk for low GH and melatonin. Sleep and GH are critical pieces for fat loss. It is also necessary to avoid eating too close to bedtime. If you consume food right before bed, you also impair this natural cool-down mechanism.

Abdominal obesity in postmenopausal women has been linked to low GH secretion, increased inflammatory markers, lipid dysregulation, and risk of developing cardiovascular disease. A 2007 study in the Journal of Endocrinology and Metabolism revealed that supplementing GH for 6 months induced significantly more loss of body weight from body fat and improved lipid profiles.[32]

GH and Mental Performance

In addition to maintaining an ideal body composition, growth hormone has been shown to be associated with an improvement in mental clarity, attention and memory.[33] People whose bodies naturally produce less GH have worse short-term and long-term memory, and they also tend to feel more tired and lethargic, too.[34] Those symptoms can lead to that "brain fog" feeling, where you feel

---

[32] Albert, Stewart G., and Arshag D. Mooradian. "Low-dose recombinant human growth hormone as adjuvant therapy to lifestyle modifications in the management of obesity." *The Journal of Clinical Endocrinology & Metabolism* 89.2 (2004): 695-701.

[33] Wass, John AH, and Raghava Reddy. "Growth hormone and memory." Journal of Endocrinology 207.2 (2010): 125-126.

[34] Deijen, J. B., et al. "Cognitive impairments and mood disturbances in growth hormone deficient men." *Psychoneuroendocrinology* 21.3 (1996): 313-322.

like you're just not as mentally sharp as you should be. Higher levels of GH can also help you improve your mood by increasing the levels of IGF-1 in your body.[35]

Natural Ways to Increase Growth Hormone

There are a number of ways that you can increase the amount of GH your body produces naturally. The most effective ways to help your body produce more GH are:

1. Practice intermittent fasting: Intermittent fasting (IF) does many amazing things for your body (and we'll discuss IF in greater detail later in the book). One of those amazing things is helping your body produce more GH. Scientific studies have shown that fasting helps to encourage your body to secrete more GH. And, IF is one of the easiest and safest ways to implement fasting into your lifestyle. (But, always check with your doctor before beginning an IF regime.)[36]

2. Lose fat: There is a strong correlation between the amount of fat you have on your body and the amount of GH your body makes. [37] This is particularly true for abdominal fat, which is very strongly associated with the amount of GH produced. People who have higher amounts of abdominal fat (and overall body fat) produce significantly less GH. So, if you want your body to produce more GH, work to lose more fat. (Following what I teach in this book will help you do just

---

[35] Lašaitė, Lina, et al. "Psychological functioning after growth hormone therapy in adult growth hormone deficient patients: endocrine and body composition correlates." *Medicina* 40.8 (2004): 740-744.

[36] Ho, Klan Y., et al. "Fasting enhances growth hormone secretion and amplifies the complex rhythms of growth hormone secretion in man." *The Journal of clinical investigation* 81.4 (1988): 968-975.

[37] Clasey, Jody L., et al. "Abdominal visceral fat and fasting insulin are important predictors of 24-hour GH release independent of age, gender, and other physiological factors." *The Journal of Clinical Endocrinology & Metabolism* 86.8 (2001): 3845-3852.

that!)

3. Get your sleep: Your body also doesn't produce as much GH when you don't sleep well.[38] And, since most GH is secreted while you're sleeping, it's important to make sure you're getting quality sleep every night. Follow the tips listed above (under "Habits to Increase Melatonin") to help fall asleep faster and stay asleep longer.

4. Incorporate high-intensity exercise: High-intensity interval training (HIIT) is not only an incredibly effective way to burn fat, but it's also a great way to increase your GH levels, too. Even 10 minutes of exercise can stimulate your body to produce more GH.[39]

5. Cryotherapy: Cryotherapy is becoming very popular in some circles. In most cases, you'll stand in a cryotherapy chamber, and you'll be surrounded by very cold air. It's often used to help reduce inflammation throughout the body, making it very popular among athletes, as well as people with chronic inflammatory diseases. There's some evidence that cryotherapy may help your body produce more GH.[40] And, the reduction in inflammation from a cryotherapy session can cause many health benefits.

6. Contrast showers: If you do not have access to cryotherapy, try contrast showers. Start with the shower on hot for 1 minute then switch it to as cold as you can tolerate for 10-30 seconds. Alternate back and forth 5 times, but make sure to end on cold (sorry).

---

[38] Honda, Yutaka, et al. "Growth hormone secretion during nocturnal sleep in normal subjects." *The Journal of Clinical Endocrinology & Metabolism* 29.1 (1969): 20-29.

[39] Felsing, Nancy E., J. A. Brasel, and Dan M. Cooper. "Effect of low and high intensity exercise on circulating growth hormone in men." *The Journal of Clinical Endocrinology & Metabolism* 75.1 (1992): 157-162.

[40] Grasso, D., et al. "Salivary steroid hormone response to whole-body cryotherapy in elite rugby players." *Journal of biological regulators and homeostatic agents* 28.2 (2014): 291-300.

7. Supplements: Certain supplements may also help the body secrete more GH. These supplements are:

    - Arginine[41]
    - Beta-alanine[42]
    - Creatine[43]
    - Glutamine[44]
    - Glycine[45]
    - L-dopa[46]
    - Melatonin[47]
    - Ornithine[48]

---

[41] Alba-Roth, Julia, et al. "Arginine stimulates growth hormone secretion by suppressing endogenous somatostatin secretion." *The Journal of Clinical Endocrinology & Metabolism* 67.6 (1988): 1186-1189.

[42] Hoffman, J., et al. "β-Alanine and the hormonal response to exercise." *International journal of sports medicine* 29.12 (2008): 952-958.

[43] Schedel, J. M., et al. "Acute creatine loading enhances human growth hormon secretion." *Journal of sports medicine and physical fitness* 40.4 (2000): 336.

[44] Welbourne, Tomas C. "Increased plasma bicarbonate and growth hormone after an oral glutamine load." *The American journal of clinical nutrition* 61.5 (1995): 1058-1061.

[45] Kasai, Kikuo, Masami Kobayashi, and Shin-Ichi Shimoda. "Stimulatory effect of glycine on human growth hormone secretion." *Metabolism-Clinical and Experimental* 27.2 (1978): 201-208.

[46] Kansal, Prakash C., et al. "The effect of L-dopa on plasma growth hormone, insulin, and thyroxine." *The Journal of Clinical Endocrinology & Metabolism* 34.1 (1972): 99-105.

[47] Valcavi, Roberto, et al. "Melatonin stimulates growth hormone secretion through pathways other than the growth hormone-releasing hormone." *Clinical endocrinology* 39.2 (1993): 193-199.

[48] Demura, Shinichi, et al. "The effect of L-ornithine hydrochloride ingestion on human growth hormone secretion after strength

training." *Advances in Bioscience and Biotechnology* 1.01 (2010): 7.

CHAPTER EIGHT

Mind Your Mitochondria —
The Secret to Lasting Energy

IF YOU CAN REMEMBER BACK TO HIGH SCHOOL BIOLOGY CLASS, YOUR MITOCHONDRIA ARE THE POWERHOUSE ORGANELLES WITHIN YOUR CELLS. You can think of them as little engines that take "fuel" from stored fat or food and combine it with oxygen to ignite a "spark" to power our cells. Another way to look at it is your mitochondria take the calories from food and convert them into a molecule called adenosine triphosphate (ATP) that your cells use for energy.

When we consume calories, our endocrine system acts as a bank account. It designates the foods we eat as "spending money," or sends them to our "savings account." All of that saved energy ultimately ends up as fat on your butt, hips, abdomen, and thighs.

The function of the mitochondria is important to fat loss for this reason. Fit individuals have increased mitochondrial function, while obese and insulin-resistant individuals have not only fewer mitochondria, but the ones they do have are sluggish and function poorly.

Obese people also have less oxygen reaching their mitochondria, and remember, oxygen is needed to create ATP or energy from the foods we eat or from our fat stores. Instead of a brightly lit fire within those mitochondria, the overweight individuals' fire smolders from lack of oxygen. That means fat burning may come to a halt, or at the very least be far less efficient. On the other hand, because mitochondria require oxygen, you can imagine the negative impact of poor, inefficient breathing techniques.

Creating more of an issue, the lack of oxygen triggers inflammation, further hampering fat burning and insulin resistance. Inflammation can misdirect metabolism into a state of increased sugar burning at the expense of fat burning, which is certainly not ideal for weight loss. The end result is not only a sluggish metabolism and difficulty losing weight, but also very low energy and intense cravings for high-fat, high-carb foods to provide any sort of boost to get through the day. It's a double whammy for weight gain. Addressing inflammation is often at the core of my prescription. Consume a diet with a focus on plants and clean meat sources. I recommend a paleo-style diet to the majority of my patients and use anti-inflammatory products like curcumin, resveratrol, Boswellia, ginger, and proteolytic enzymes.

Factors that Affect Mitochondrial Function

Mitochondria are organelles found in large numbers in most cells. They play a key role in the biochemical processes of cellular respiration and energy production. (Cellular respiration is simply how cells use oxygen to create energy for the cell, not how cells breathe.) This is the reason why mitochondria are referred to as the power plant or energy plant of the cell, or even the furnace of the cell.

If you want your body to burn more fat so you can change your body composition, it's going to happen in your mitochondria. This is because your mitochondria take fat and convert it to energy through beta oxidation. The first step occurs when L-carnitine, an amino acid, transports fatty acids across the mitochondrial membrane. Once the mitochondria receive the fatty acids, they take them through the Krebs cycle, using oxygen and other cofactors to produce energy. So, if you are low in L-carnitine, fatty acids will not be transported into the mitochondria to be burned as fuel, hindering fat loss.

If you are anemic, red blood cells will not carry oxygen very well. That means less oxygen will get to your cells for your mitochondria to use. Thus, your cells won't effectively produce ATP for energy. Remember, your mitochondria need to burn fat molecules if you're going to lose fat on your body. So, if you've been struggling to shed fat, you should make sure you're not anemic. The oxygen requirement is another reason why deep, proper breathing is so important.

In addition, if fats are not being brought into the cell and into the mitochondria efficiently, acidic byproducts back up. If this occurs, medical professionals can see increases in clusters of markers that indicate that your body isn't producing enough of important transport molecules, cofactors, or getting enough oxygen.

Tests for Mitochondrial Health

When working with patients with chronic energy depletion and fatigue, it is important to take a complete health history of stressors, infections, respiratory illness, peripheral vascular disease, and cardiovascular health. In addition, I recommend running basic blood chemistry such as a complete blood count, ferritin levels, iron, and iron saturation, and thorough thyroid function testing to rule out whether they have significant internal disorder. Integrative testing is also often required, which may include genetics, adrenal stress indexes, hormone testing, and organic acid testing. Adrenal testing is beneficial, as an overactive stress response or depleted adrenal function can contribute to chronic fatigue.

The organic acids panel or metabolic profile looks at the unique biochemistry of the individual in critical domains, including how your cells make energy. The DUTCH plus test now includes six organic acid tests (OATs), including markers for vitamin B12 (methylmalonate), vitamin B6 (xanthurenate), glutathione (pyroglutamate), dopamine (homovanillate), norepinephrine/epinephrine (vanilmandelate), and serotonin (5-hydroxyindoleacetate). The results of organic acid testing can indicate whether you are an efficient converter of carbohydrates, fats and proteins into energy (ATP). The organic acids test also reveals an individual's unique sufficiency or insufficiency of key vitamin and mineral cofactors. It will also tell us a great deal about neurotransmitter metabolites, oxidative stress, toxic exposure, efficacy of detoxification pathways, and bacterial and fungal overgrowth.

Anemia

Low iron, or anemia, is common cause of fatigue and unfortunately conventional practitioners wait for overt shifts in markers. You can be functionally anemic and present with symptoms like fatigue, hair loss, shortness of breath, and reduced exercise tolerance. And, you can experience these symptoms for a long time before you have an overtly low red blood cell count. This is where integrative testing is important. Just because you are within "normal" range does not mean you are optimal. Normal range of ferritin, the storage form of iron, is between 10 and 220, but women who have ferritin levels of less than 50-70 usually have clinical symptomatology of iron deficiency.

If anemia due to low B12 or iron is contributing to the fatigue, it is important to start with diet. Looking to the root cause is very important, and supplementing with nutraceuticals is only a temporary bandage. Ask the hard questions. Is there a reason why you are not absorbing iron, or are you simply not getting enough folate or B12 in your diet? If you are consuming adequate amount of these nutrients but your levels are low, ask why you are not absorbing them. Is there an underlying gut issue such as leaky gut, IBS, or gastrointestinal (GI) mucosal issue?

Lastly, if you are supplementing, instead of using standard ferrous sulfate (which is not well absorbed and can cause nausea and constipation), use a ferrous bisglycinate chelate such as Ferrochel by Designs for Health. Ferrochel, produced from Albion Chelated Minerals, is better absorbed, and does not have gastric side effects. When considering supplementing with B12 and/or folate, ensure you are using methylated folate (5-MTHF) and a methylated cobalamin, not a cyanocobalamin.

Nutrients and the Mitochondria

The world we live in today is riddled with environmental and food toxins. Pesticides, chemical fertilizers, radiation, smog, smoke and preservatives, to name a few, have damaging effects on all of our cells. Exposure to these toxins can encourage harmful free radicals to accumulate in our bodies. Free radicals create a destructive chain reaction in our cells, leading to compromised cell function that robs us of our health and vitality.

As we age, the ongoing exposure to free radicals causes deterioration of the mitochondria. This deprives other cellular components of energy, and subsequently accelerates their destruction, causing them to function less efficiently. Supporting healthy mitochondria and energy production helps optimize energy levels, while protecting cells from destruction and aging. Additionally, healthy mitochondria within the brain cells can help support optimal brain health and wellness.

So how can you take care of your mitochondria and make sure you are doing everything you can to support their function? Here are key nutrients for mitochondrial health that you should make sure you're getting:

- Coenzyme Q10 – A critical component of energy (ATP)

production
- L-carnitine and pantethine – Aid in shuttling fats from the bloodstream into the mitochondria, where they are converted into energy
- Alpha lipoic acid and B vitamins – Assist various enzymes that function in the energy-producing pathways of the body
- Malic and succinic acids – Specific components of the Krebs cycle, one of the main energy-producing pathways in the mitochondria
- Creatine – Supports additional energy production; necessary for healthy mitochondria
- Resveratrol and curcumin – Botanicals that encourage the natural production of additional mitochondria within the cell
- Pyrroloquinoline quinone (PQQ) - a water-soluble vitamin-like compound found in green tea, green peppers, parsley, kiwi, papaya, and other foods. It is a potent antioxidant and protects the mitochondria from oxidative damage. PQQ also triggers mitochondrial biogenesis, increasing the number of mitochondria in the body.

If you choose to take a supplement to improve the health of your mitochondria, it's important to take a supplement that provides the nutrients your mitochondria need in the right ways. My mitochondrial support supplements of choice are Mitochondrial NRG, PQQ, CoQ10, and Resveratrol. These supplements may be beneficial for:

- Healthy energy levels
- Aiding exercise intolerance
- Improved athletic performance
- Helping to alleviate post-exercise muscle soreness
- Efficient fat burning
- Healthy weight management
- Mental clarity
- Improving overall cellular and tissue vitality and health

Exercise and Mitochondria

Remember that your mitochondria produce the energy your cells need to function. This is particularly true when you're doing high-energy activities like exercise. The good news is you can improve the health of your mitochondria when you exercise. Exercise stimulates the production of more mitochondria,[49] and those mitochondria have more of the enzymes and components that allow them to create more energetic molecules (ATP) from carbohydrates and fats.[50] In short, exercise helps you create mitochondria that are more efficient at burning fat, and it helps you make more of them, too.

What type of exercise should you do if you want to produce mitochondria that are incredible fat burners? High burst, high intensity aerobic activity is an extremely effective way to stimulate your muscle cells to produce more and better mitochondria.[51] This type of exercise works by increasing mitochondrial transcription factors, which are responsible for signaling the production of more production of mitochondria.[52] You'll find some suggestions for exercise that will help you burn more fat in Chapter 14.

---

[49] Morgan, T. E., et al. "Effects of long-term exercise on human muscle mitochondria." *Muscle metabolism during exercise*. Springer, Boston, MA, 1971. 87-95.

[50] Gollnick, Philip D., and Douglas W. King. "Effect of exercise and training on mitochondria of rat skeletal muscle." *American Journal of Physiology-Legacy Content* 216.6 (1969): 1502-1509.

[51] Gibala, Martin J., and Sean L. McGee. "Metabolic adaptations to short-term high-intensity interval training: a little pain for a lot of gain?" *Exercise and sport sciences reviews* 36.2 (2008): 58-63.

[52] Little, Jonathan P., et al. "An acute bout of high-intensity interval training increases the nuclear abundance of PGC-1α and activates mitochondrial biogenesis in human skeletal muscle." *American Journal of Physiology-Regulatory, Integrative and Comparative Physiology* 300.6 (2011): R1303-R1310.

CHAPTER NINE

Digestion and Gut Health

S O FAR IN THIS BOOK, WE'VE SPENT A LOT OF TIME
FOCUSING ON THE HORMONES THAT ARE PRODUCED
IN DIFFERENT AREAS OF THE BODY AND HOW THOSE
HORMONES CAN IMPACT WEIGHT AND FAT LOSS. In this
chapter, I'd like to focus on one of the body's major processes,
digestion, and how the health of your digestive system can impact
your hormones.

For a long time, many medical professionals ignored or minimized
the importance of gut health. But over the past few decades, more and
more research has shown that your gut health is incredibly important,
affecting everything from immune function to mental health and
more.

A calorie is not just a calorie; they are not created equally and here
is the reason why. The calories that we consume can have
dramatically different effects on our gut microbiome (the microbes
that live in the gut) and thus our hormones and metabolism. Even the
speed in which you consume food, the position you eat in (sitting vs
on the go), the time of day you eat, the amount of fibre, alcohol,

fructose, and the combination of foods can influence what makes up your gut microbiome and how your body processes calories.

For instance, fructose is processed differently than glucose. Fructose blunts satiety signals, alters intestinal bacteria, and increases levels of the appetite-stimulating hormone ghrelin.[53] To make matters worse, fructose stimulates the reward centers in the brain, creating food addictions.[54] Lastly, fructose has been shown to be able to widen the spaces between intestinal cells, increasing the risk of absorbing bacterial endotoxins which then promote inflammation.[55]

The Estrobolome

Back in Chapter 5, we took a look at the hormone estrogen. Estrogen is mostly synthesized in the ovaries, but many other glands and tissues produce estrogen in small and moderate amounts. For example, adipose tissue is an important source of estrogen in both men and women and because our fat tissue is metabolically active, the more you have, the more estrogen it will produce. Last but not least, our adrenal glands also produce some estrogen.

Estrogen starts to cause problems when it becomes unbalanced in the body. These imbalances can become particularly acute if you're exposed to estrogen and estrogen-mimicking chemicals in your environment. Xenobiotics (chemicals that resemble estrogen) and endocrine disruptors are becoming increasingly common in our environments. These chemicals include things like pharmaceuticals (like the oral contraceptive pill), herbicides, pesticides, heavy metals,

---

[53] Vos, Miriam B., and Craig J. McClain. "Fructose takes a toll." *Hepatology* 50.4 (2009): 1004-1006.

[54] Purnell, Jonathan Q., and Damien A. Fair. "Fructose ingestion and cerebral, metabolic, and satiety responses." *Jama* 309.1 (2013): 85-86.

[55] Spruss, Astrid, and Ina Bergheim. "Dietary fructose and intestinal barrier: potential risk factor in the pathogenesis of nonalcoholic fatty liver disease." *The Journal of nutritional biochemistry* 20.9 (2009): 657-662.

and plasticizers. And, the worst part is, they're found everywhere, from your drinking water to your skincare products.

So, what can you do to keep your estrobolome happy? First, limit your exposure to environmental estrogens and estrogen mimics as much as possible. Eat organic foods and use clean body and skincare products. Also, remember that your liver is key when it comes to removing excess estrogen from your body. Go back and reread Chapter 2 and 5 to learn more about how you can support your liver and help it metabolize hormones properly so your body can maintain proper hormone balance.

From the liver, your body's excess estrogen is secreted through bile. It passes through your gall bladder into your intestines. There, it meets up with all sorts of beneficial bacteria that live in your intestine that are part of your gut microbiome. The microbes in your intestine are incredibly important to your health, and there are a lot of them. (The number of microbe cells actually outnumbers human cells in the intestine!)

Your gut bacteria can actually modify the excreted estrogen in the bile through a process called conjugation. This makes the estrogen active again, and it can be reabsorbed and circulated throughout the body. (This process is called enterohepatic recirculation, which simply means that hormones go from your liver down to your gut, then back up to your liver.) If those hormones get recirculated, it can really throw your hormone balance out of whack.

That's why we want good bacteria in the gut to modify the excess estrogens in the bile so that they'll be excreted in feces, not reabsorbed. You should be doing everything you can to support these good bacteria to keep your hormones in balance. To keep them healthy, you can consume fermented foods like kimchi, sauerkraut, or pickles. You may also ask your doctor whether you should be taking a probiotic supplement to help keep your gut flora healthy.

You should also make sure that your good gut bacteria have the food they need to thrive. The good news is that it's easy to get them what they need. You may have heard of prebiotics, which is the food and nutrients that help your good bacteria grow. Prebiotics are simply fibre-rich foods that support the growth of good bacteria. You can get prebiotics by including lots of plants in your diet. You can also supplement with psyllium husk, flax seeds, and other fibre-rich products. I personally in addition to a high fiber diet, add supplemental fibers in a rotating fashion to make sure I am giving my gut bacteria the prebiotics they need to thrive. Examples include Biota Balance (the fiber product I created), PaleoFiber, Daily Cleanse, and the delicious Coco Fibre Bars.

Leaky Gut and Hypothyroidism: The Connection

If you have been diagnosed with hypothyroidism, you were most likely told that it is a genetic condition, that you will have to take a medication for the rest of your life, and that is about all that can be done for you. I would also bet you were never asked about your digestion or symptoms of adrenal fatigue such as stress and cravings. Taking this a step further, I would bet that your doctor never mentioned that your gut and your thyroid were connected in any way.

In conventional medicine, an endocrinologist is the expert in hormones, and gut health is left for the specialty of gastroenterologists. But, there is a connection between the adrenals, thyroid, and gut! We need to address all pieces of the puzzle if you want the best chance to restore the function of your thyroid.

Leaky Gut and Hypothyroidism

Hashimoto's, or autoimmune thyroid disease, is the number one cause of hypothyroidism in North America. While not all causes of hypothyroidism are well understood, we do know that if you have an autoimmune condition, then your immune system is not behaving as it should.

And where is 70-80% of your immune system located? Your gut!

Your digestive system is essentially a long tube from your mouth to your rectum that is lined with a semipermeable layer of cells. This separation acts like a strainer to allow only some key nutrients to be absorbed and passed. At the same time, the intestinal lining should keep harmful proteins from entering your body. When our small intestines get damaged, like in a "leaky gut," the straining, absorption, and secretion functions become impaired. That allows infectious agents, food particles, and other proteins to make their way through the lining of the intestine. Exposure to these "non-self" proteins or antigens stimulates the immune system to produce antibodies.

Producing antibodies is normally a good thing! It tags the foreign particle to be removed from the body. However, the issue lies in a term called "molecular mimicry." In molecular mimicry, the non-self protein that has been tagged for destruction resembles an amino acid sequence of self proteins, AKA body tissues. When this happens, your immune system can mistake your tissues as foreign and begin to attack them, in addition to causing inflammation in the body.

Over time, after repeat exposure, the body will respond by creating antibodies, which can set off a cascade of autoimmune destruction of the thyroid tissue — resulting in Hashimoto's and eventually hypothyroidism.

Potential Causes of Leaky Gut

So, what causes leaky gut? We've only realized the importance of leaky gut for a handful of years, so there hasn't been enough time to thoroughly study it scientifically to learn why it happens. But, there is some evidence to show that the following foods and chemicals may contribute to leaky gut:

- GMO Foods
- Prescription Medications: NSAIDs & Antibiotics
- Alcohol & Caffeine

- Mold Exposure
- Gluten & Dairy
- Food Sensitivities
- Processed Sugar
- Cosmetic Products
- Harsh Household Chemicals
- Contaminated Water
- Packaged Food & Teflon
- Emotional & Mental Stress

If you're working to heal your leaky gut, work to avoid these as much as possible.

Common Symptoms of Leaky Gut

You may be thinking, "I don't have any gut issues. What does this have to do with my thyroid and other hormones?" Leaky gut symptoms can affect the whole body, and everyone responds differently. In fact, it is possible to have sensitivities, dysbiosis, other gut conditions, and even celiac disease without any obvious gut symptoms.

While many do experience GI symptoms such as gas, bloating, diarrhea, and intolerances or sensitivities, others may find their thyroid is impacted first. Leaky gut can also cause issues in these areas of the body:

- Sinus & mouth: colds, food sensitivities
- Brain: depression, ADHD, anxiety, headache
- Skin: rashes, rosacea, psoriasis, eczema, acne
- Thyroid: Hashimoto's, Graves hypothyroid, metabolism
- Colon: constipation, diarrhea, IBD, IBS
- Joints: rheumatoid arthritis, fibromyalgia & chronic fatigue
- Adrenal fatigue

As our gut health goes undetected or ignored, sometimes for years or decades, the gut lining is not performing at its best due to intestinal damage. For some patients, the diagnosis of autoimmune disease is their first sign that something is wrong in the gut.

This is why I like to focus on the gut when treating autoimmune disease. But beyond autoimmune conditions, your gut does support your thyroid in many other ways, too.

How Your Gut Affects Thyroid Hormones

Remember that your body produces inactive T4 that needs to converted into the active version, T3. T3 is responsible for your energy, metabolism, body heat, and much more. T4 is primarily converted to T3 in the liver and kidneys, and about 20% of your thyroid hormone conversion takes place in the gut. Thus, a healthy gut flora plays an important role in making sure you get the appropriate amount of T3. Peripheral conversion of thyroid hormone is a vital process in ensuring you are receiving adequate thyroid hormone because T4 accounts for about 95% of all hormone produced by your thyroid, T3 being the other 5% that requires peripheral conversion. If your gut is not functioning optimally, you can experience symptoms of hypothyroidism, even if your thyroid is healthy.

In addition to a healthy gut microbiome you also need adequate stomach acid for a healthy thyroid. If you have low stomach acid, you will not be able to break down and thus absorb the many nutrients necessary for thyroid function that you consume. Taking Betaine HCl, or digestive enzymes containing HCl, will take the pressure off the digestive system. Digestive enzymes will also help to break down proteins that may be negatively triggering the immune system through a process called molecular mimicry. Ask your Functional Medicine Doctor or Naturopath about adding this to your regimen.

Inflammation also plays a part in how your gut can affect your thyroid hormones. Inflammation in our bodies increases our risk for a variety of chronic health concerns. Healthy gut flora will inhibit pro-inflammatory cytokines like IL-6, TNF-alpha, NFK-b and upregulate anti-inflammatory cytokines like IL-10.

The bottom line is that when our gut microbiomes are not happy, inflammation goes up. When inflammation increases, cortisol, our stress hormone, follows. It is cortisol that causes issues to our thyroid because it down-regulates, or reduces the conversion of inactive T4 to active T3.

In addition, constipation can create hormone imbalances that lead to increased levels of estrogen. As estrogen levels increase, so do proteins aimed at keeping the hormone bound. The same mechanisms that lead to excess estrogen being bound can cause thyroid hormone to also become unavailable.

Low levels of circulating thyroid hormone can cause impaired gut motility and constipation, which can perpetuate the cycle of hormone imbalance. This is another example of how gut function is crucial to having adequate levels of thyroid hormone available.

Healing Your Gut

There are a variety of approaches to treat autoimmune and thyroid conditions. In my opinion, you cannot look at the thyroid in isolation. You must also heal your gut if you want to optimize thyroid health, balance hormones, and reduce autoimmunity.

When developing treatment protocols, I take a holistic approach that is unique and specific to each individual's needs. Functional and comprehensive lab testing is valuable in conjunction with your story, to ensure proper treatment. While many physicians test TSH alone, this is not enough to understand the complete picture. TSH, free T4, free T3, thyroid antibodies, and reverse T3 should all be considered if you are presenting with symptoms of thyroid disease.

With that in mind, here are three basic steps I take with patients looking to heal their guts and improve thyroid health. Again, I highly recommend you find a practitioner who is trained and able to work with you to get to the root cause of your symptoms prior to starting any course of treatment.

Step 1: Remove Inflammatory Triggers

Food Sensitivities — A free way to identify possible food sensitivities is to remove the potential irritant for 3-6 weeks. This is called an elimination diet. Top food allergens to remove are gluten, dairy, eggs, corn, soy, nuts, and beans/legumes (including peanuts). After the elimination phase, reintroduce foods one by one over a three-day period. For support in completing an elimination diet consider joining my 10-day challenge where I make the process easy.

Over-exercising — While I love to see patients moving their bodies, over-exercising is a source of stress on our bodies and creates inflammation. If paired with undereating, it's a recipe for disaster. This is why it is so important to eat the right foods, at the right times for the right reasons.

Chronic Stress — As I mentioned above, chronic stress can alter your gut microbiome and creates inflammation. Stress or cortisol is a major hormone that impacts the HPA-axis (hypothalamic-pituitary-adrenal). If you throw your HPA axis out of whack, pretty much all the hormones in your body will be affected.

Unnecessary Medications — Medications such as NSAIDs, unnecessary antibiotics, birth control, antidepressants and proton pump inhibitors (PPIs) may negatively affect gut health. Do not discontinue any medications before talking with your doctor.

Bacteria, Yeast, Parasites — Ask your doctor if gut dysbiosis or overgrowth of bacteria, yeast, or parasites may be contributing to chronic gut complaints or thyroid issues. Testing is an option to see if any critters are living happily undetected.

Step 2: Nourish the Gut Lining

Amino Acids — Amino acids proline, glycine, and glutamine are critical to gut health. Proline, which is high in bone broth, supports collagen and helps to tighten the tight junctions that have become leaky. Glycine supports detoxification of your liver and cellular pathways. L-glutamine is used as fuel by intestinal cells to heal the gut lining.

Coconut Oil — Coconut oil is amazing for leaky gut due to its antimicrobial effects. Coconut can be used in smoothies and cooking, as well as in your coffee.

Curcumin — Turmeric is an amazing herb that is beneficial to your overall health and reduces inflammation.

Zinc Carnosine — Zinc and vitamin C increase healing time and boost immune function.

Vitamin D — The Vitamin D receptor plays a role in intestinal barrier integrity as well as it enhances healing of the colonic epithelium. Therefore, a deficiency in vitamin D may compromise the barrier and increase risk of damage and inflammation.

Digestive Enzymes — Digestive enzymes are the catalyst to break down nutrients that we consume. Digestive enzymes can help heal leaky gut by taking the stress of the GI tract. They help to break down difficult-to-digest protein and sugars like gluten, casein and lactose.

Betaine HCl and Pepsin — If you have low stomach acid you will not be able to break down and thus absorb the nutrients you consume. Taking Betaine HCl, like the digestive enzymes, will take the pressure off the digestive system. Ask your doctor about adding this to your regimen.

Berries — Not only are berries a rich source of antioxidants but they are also high in flavonoids, which reduce intestinal inflammation and protect the gut. Berries are an easily digestible form of fibre and are a healthy way to satisfy sugar cravings.

Step 3: Rebalance the microbiome

Fermented Vegetables — Diets rich in fermented foods are key to your health regime. Other strategies include constant exposure to soil-based organisms by spending time outdoors, being around animals, and eaten locally-grown foods.

Probiotics — Taking targeted strains for your unique symptom picture is the best way to approach probiotics. Gut microbial diversity is extremely important. Ask your doctor about strains that would be best for you. *Saccharomyces boulardi* is one strain that has been shown to protect against pathogens, increase beneficial immune response, protect gastrointestinal barrier function, and promote enzymatic activity so you can better absorb nutrients from your food!

Note: If your digestive symptoms get worse or you experience extreme gas or bloating when probiotic foods or supplements are introduced, I recommend reducing or eliminating probiotics and talking with your doctor about SIBO testing or fructose intolerance.

Getting to the root of your gut issues is an important step toward healing your thyroid and your health. That's why I am passionate about holistic care, and understand the importance of conventional and functional lab testing and can interpret those tests in conjunction with your story. I want to help you feel your best so you can go on to do everything you were meant to do.

CHAPTER TEN

Blood Sugar, Insulin Resistance, and Glucagon

IN ORDER TO UNDERSTAND WHY YOU'RE STRUGGLING TO LOSE FAT, IT'S INCREDIBLY IMPORTANT TO UNDERSTAND HOW THE HORMONE INSULIN AFFECTS YOUR BODY. Insulin is one of the seven key hormones that can have a huge *impact* on your weight and how much fat your body stores. Luckily, when you eat the right foods at the right time, you can work with your body's natural insulin levels to burn more fat and support the proper levels of other hormones in your body.

Insulin resistance has become an epidemic in North American culture. It is contributing to many of the chronic health problems we see today, including obesity, type 2 diabetes, and heart disease. It is also associated with high blood pressure, high cholesterol, thyroid problems, muscle loss, fat gain, fatty liver, breast cancer, endometrial cancer, and other cancers as well. And, insulin resistance has even been implicated in Alzheimer's disease, with some professionals referring to Alzheimer's as type 3 diabetes.

Insulin is a hormone that is secreted by the pancreas. It has a direct impact on your body's blood sugar levels by affecting how quickly your body's cells absorb sugar from the bloodstream. If your blood sugar is too high, insulin signals the body to store that excess sugar in your liver in the form of glycogen, where it can later be broken down and turned back into sugar when needed.

If you are the type to graze on foods all day or if you are consuming a high carbohydrate diet, chances are your insulin levels are high. Elevated insulin has negative consequences such as inflammation and increased risk of developing type 2 diabetes, making weight loss difficult. Insulin also impacts sex hormones like estrogen and progesterone. If insulin is high, it stimulates estrogen and lowers progesterone as well as blocks the progesterone receptors. This can manifest as infertility, PCOS, endometriosis, resistant weight loss, PMS, and other hormone health conditions.

Glycemic Index and Glycemic Load

In technical terms, the glycemic index (GI) of foods is determined by how they immediately influence blood sugar levels in the body when we eat them. So, what exactly does that mean? Think of a water balloon. If you were to drop a balloon from a high building, the balloon would be broken quickly on impact and a "gush" of water would be released. In the body, foods with a high glycemic index are quickly digested and broken down resulting in a high, fast blood sugar response.

If you were to take the same balloon and drop it from a low height and a stone pierced a small hole in the balloon the water would dribble out. Similar to this balloon, foods with low glycemic indexes are slow to digest and breakdown. This results in a slow but gradual release of glucose into the bloodstream.

A GI of 70 or more is high, a GI of 56 to 69 inclusive is medium, and a GI of 55 or less is low.

For memory's sake, we can think of high glycemic index foods as "bursters" or "gushers" and low glycemic index foods as "drippers."

The glycemic load (GL) is also often used to categorize foods and gives a fuller picture than does glycemic index alone. A glycemic index tells you how rapidly a carbohydrate turns into sugar, but it doesn't tell you how much of that carbohydrate is in a serving of a certain food. To know the full effect on blood sugar it is important to know the glycemic index and glycemic load.

For example, the carbohydrate in watermelon has a high glycemic index, BUT watermelon doesn't have a lot of sugar per serving, so the glycemic load is low. To calculate glycemic load the quality of a carbohydrate in a given food (glycemic index) is multiplied by the amount of carbohydrate in a serving of that food. By knowing both values we have a better indication on how a carbohydrate food will affect blood sugar.

Which of these is more important for people like diabetics, or those who want to lose weight, to consider?

Knowing both GI and GL allows a nine-component grid to be created low GL with low, medium, and high GI, medium GL with low, medium, and high GI, and high GL with low and medium high GI. Careful and accurate interpretation of glycemic effect of food therefore necessitates an understanding of both glucose load and glycemic index.

The type of foods we consume dictate what your body is going to burn as fuel to survive and what it is going to store as body fat. The aim of weight loss is to build muscle and release body fat. Low glycemic foods are beneficial in weight loss as the body tends to use fat for fuel instead of relying on muscle. Foods that have a low glycemic index are also advantageous for weight loss because they fell to make you feel full faster and for longer.

Is it possible for foods to be high in one, but not the other?

Actually yes!

The carbohydrate in watermelon, for example, has a pretty high GI (about 72), but there isn't a lot of it, so watermelon's glycemic load is relatively low.

To calculate glycemic load, glycemic index is divided by 100 multiplied by its available carbohydrate content (i.e. carbohydrates minus fibre) in grams.

Example: A 100-gram serving of watermelon has about eight grams of available carbohydrate.

Its glycemic load, therefore is 72/100*8 =5.04, rounded to 5.

A GL of 20 or more is high, a GL of 11 to 19 inclusive is medium, and a GL of 10 or less is low.

Thus, watermelon has a high glycemic index, but because few carbohydrates are available per serving, the glycemic load is low. Careful and accurate interpretation of glycemic effect of food therefore necessitates an understanding of both glucose load and glycemic index.

How can people easily keep track of and monitor GI and GL?

Take advantage of technology. There are many apps out there that track GI and GL quickly and efficiently. Some examples are "Glyndex," "Glycemic Index and Glycemic Load," "Glycemic Index & Load Diet Aid," and "Low GI Diet Tracker." It is all about first finding an app that is compatible with your device, but most importantly, one that you will actually use.

Is Stress the Missing Component to Insulin Resistance?

There is new evidence to suggest diet and exercise are not the only factors we can target to improve insulin resistance and diabetes.

Evidence shows cortisol directly triggers a physiological hyperglycemia and psychological stress is therefore identified as a chief determinant in the development of visceral adiposity and insulin insensitivity. In one study, stress from work predicted 125% increased risk metabolic syndrome (three major events versus none over a 14-year period).[56]

Your Cycle and Insulin Sensitivity

Your menstrual cycle and changes in hormones can affect your sensitivity to insulin. When your body's cells are exposed to estrogen, they also become more sensitive to insulin. Conversely, if your body's natural estrogen levels begin to wane, your cells may become insulin resistant. That is why many women struggle with insulin resistance as they go through menopause.

Insulin sensitivity will be highest when your estrogen levels are also highest, which occurs during the follicular phase of your cycle, which is roughly the first half of your cycle. During this time, you can work out harder because fuel will naturally be more available to your muscles. Your body and cells will also be able to process carbs more easily due to the increased insulin sensitivity.

During the second half of your cycle, the luteal phase, your body's estrogen levels begin to dip as progesterone levels rise. Your cells will be less sensitive to insulin, which means it may be time to cut back on the carbs. You might consider experimenting with a low carb or ketogenic plan during this time to compensate for the reduced insulin sensitivity.

Go back and review Chapter 5 for more information on how to use your workouts and diet alongside your menstrual cycle to lose more fat.

---

[56] Chandola, T. "Chronic Stress At Work And The Metabolic Syndrome: Prospective Study". BMJ 332.7540 (2006): 521-525. Web.

How Can Blood Sugar and Insulin Resistance Affect Your Hormones?

Insulin resistance means your cells can't absorb the extra blood glucose your body keeps generating from the food you eat, and your liver converts the glucose into fat. Insulin resistance causes weight gain and sugar addiction.

When you consume too much sugar over a long period of time, it results in hyperinsulinemia (high insulin in the blood). Your pancreas is producing the insulin, but the cellular uptake is not happening because of the cellular resistance. As a result, you have excess circulating insulin (hyperinsulinemia).

Hyperinsulinemia can then affect the levels of other hormones in the body, such as testosterone. Refer back to Chapter 5 (particularly the section on PCOS) to refresh your memory and learn how your blood sugar affects sex hormone levels.

Blood Sugar and Cortisol

Cortisol regulates your blood sugar, your immune function, and your blood pressure. The problem is, most of us don't regulate our cortisol. Cortisol works by releasing a quick burst of glucose into your system. This is important when you need to wake up in the morning or, say, run away from a tiger, but it's not very helpful when it comes to a busy job or financial worries.

How can you make sure your blood sugar levels are where they should be and avoid insulin resistance? Put simply, manage your cortisol. Chronically high cortisol leads to chronically-high blood sugar. Here are some of my favourite ways to keep cortisol at healthy levels:

- Consider taking a fish oil supplement
- Cut down on caffeine

- Chanting and deep breathing (great for an in-the-car relaxation session!)
- Reduce alcohol to two or three servings per week
- Eat dark chocolate (doctor's orders)
- Add Vitamin B5, B6, Magnesium or Vitamin C (I recommend Liposomal) to your daily routine

Exercise is one of the best ways to lower your blood sugar and increase your insulin sensitivity. What most people don't know is that certain types of high-impact exercise (like running) actually increase cortisol, and as a result, increase blood sugar. The following are some of my favourite ways to burn some calories and beat blood sugar.

- Yoga
- Pilates
- Power walking (just add girlfriends for an added boost of oxytocin)
- Burst or interval training

How Does Cortisol Raise Blood Glucose?

Increased Breakdown of Glycogen — In our liver, glucose molecules are strung together and stored as glycogen. The liver contains significant amounts of stored glycogen which is available for rapid release into circulation. Cortisol stimulates the breakdown of liver glycogen stores.[57]

Increased Breakdown of Fat — While this may sound positive, what actually happens is your body breaks down peripheral fat and relocates it to visceral fat cells (those under the muscle, deep in the abdomen).[58] Visceral fat is the dangerous fat around the midsection.

---

[57] "Endocrine Core Notes". Rose-hulman.edu. N.p., 2017. Web. 11 Apr. 2017.
[58] Epel ES, McEwen B, Seeman T, et al. Stress and body shape: Stress-

Its danger is related to the release of proteins and hormones that can cause inflammation, which in turn can damage arteries and enter your liver. This is why visceral fat is associated with an increased risk for cardiovascular disease markers like high triglycerides, high blood pressure, and high cholesterol.

Increased Appetite and Cravings — Because your body wants an immediate source of fuel, cortisol acts to increase appetite and cravings for high-calorie foods. Studies have demonstrated a direct association between cortisol levels and calorie intake.[59] Cortisol may directly influence appetite and cravings by binding to receptors on the hypothalamus in the brain. Cortisol also indirectly influences appetite by modulating other hormones and stress responsive factors known to stimulate appetite.

Increased Muscle Breakdown — In times of high stress, the body will break down amino acids to be converted to glucose through the process of gluconeogenesis. Cortisol is the major stress hormone that catalyzes this process. We do not want to be breaking down our muscle because this will lower our metabolic rate, making it more likely will we store fat. As a side note, collagen can be a target for spare amino acids. Chronically-elevated stress levels increase collagen breakdown which is not good for the aging process!

All the above ways that cortisol elevates blood glucose also leads to fat storage!

Other Negative Effects of Cortisol

1. **Increased Bone Breakdown** — Cortisol acts to reduce bone density by inhibiting osteoblast (bone making cells) formation

---

induced cortisol secretion is consistently greater among women with central fat. *Psychosom Med.* 2000;62(5):623-632.

[59] Epel E, Lapidus R, McEwen B, Brownell K. Stress may add bite to appetite in women: A laboratory study of stress-induced cortisol and eating behavior. *Psychoneuroendocrinology.* 2001;26(1):37-49.

and cell proliferation. This dramatically decreases bone building and lowers bone density increasing risk for osteopenia and osteoporosis.

2. **Decreased Secretory IgA** — IgA is an immunoglobulin that coats our digestive track. It has a really important role to keep us protected from gut infections and dysbiosis. Decreased secretory IgA is seen in leaky gut, as well as in chronically stressed individuals.[60] As a result of leaky gut, not only are foods not being properly broken down, they are getting through into the bloodstream. This results in food sensitivities and inflammation, which in turn further elevates cortisol.

3. **Increased Th2 Immune Response:** Our immune system response can be divided into two legs. The Th1 leg is our humeral response, and Th2 leg is our cell-mediated response. Both legs are important for protecting us in different ways and must be balanced. Chronic stress elevates the Th2 response, the antibody-producing side of our immune system, and lowers the Th1, the anti-cancer, anti-infectious side. This is not good news if you have leaky gut, because now you have more of the immunoglobins or antibodies to react with those food particles that are getting through into the blood stream.

Cortisol Impacts on the Brain:

1. **Reduced Hippocampus Size** — The hippocampus is an area in the brain which is responsible for converting short to long term memory. Chronic stress has been shown in rats to reduce hippocampus size and functioning.[61] In Alzheimer's disease,

---

[60] Phillips, Anna C., et al. "Stressful life events are associated with low secretion rates of immunoglobulin A in saliva in the middle aged and elderly." *Brain, behavior, and immunity* 20.2 (2006): 191-197.

[61] Murakami, Shuji, et al. "Chronic stress, as well as acute stress, reduces

the hippocampus is one of the areas that suffers damage. It has been hypothesized that because chronic stress damages the hippocampus, it may contribute to the development of Alzheimer's disease or short-term memory loss and disorientation.

2. **Decreased Frontal lobe activity:** The frontal lobe is important for our personality, problem solving, memory, initiation, judgement, impulse control, and social and sexual behaviour. Chronic stress reduces frontal lobe activity, which can lead to anxiety, depression, as well as difficulty with concentration and memory.[62]

As you can see, the effects of chronic stress are complex. Stress reduction is more important than ever as we are faced daily with obstacles in our environments. Stress can be from emotions, over-exercise, under eating, chronic disease, inflammation, gut imbalance, toxicity, and much more. This is why measuring your cortisol response throughout the day, as well as stress reduction, should be a part of your daily routine!

Blood Sugar and Your Diet

You should also work to change your diet. Diet may be the most obvious – and the most effective – way you can positively affect your blood sugar levels. You have to eat to live, but choosing your foods based on your body's needs can help you live a lot longer. Below are the best ways to adjust your diet in a way that keeps your blood sugar low and steady.

- Don't drink your calories: commercial juices and coffee shop

---

BDNF mRNA expression in the rat hippocampus but less robustly." *Neuroscience research* 53.2 (2005): 129-139.

[62] Arnsten, Amy FT. "Stress signalling pathways that impair prefrontal cortex structure and function." *Nature Reviews Neuroscience* 10.6 (2009): 410-422.

drinks are serious sugar bombs.

- Cut out sugar wherever possible, including artificial sweeteners.
- Add fibre. Not only will fibre keep you fuller longer, but it will also help flush toxins out of your body.

Become a whole foodist. Adding lots of fruits and vegetables to your diet doesn't just add vitamins and minerals – it keeps your carbohydrate count low and your fibre high.

CHAPTER ELEVEN

Genetics

W HILE YOUR GENES ARE NOT YOUR DESTINY, HOW YOUR GENES ARE EXPRESSED DOES IMPACT YOUR VULNERABILITY TO NOT ONLY DISEASE, BUT ALSO TO BEING OVERWEIGHT. So, what is this mysterious "X factor" that has the ability to manipulate our genetic inheritance and create health rather than illness?

It is called epigenetics, the study of gene expression. As it turns out, genes can be turned "on" or "off" through a process called methylation, a biochemical process that occurs within our body. Factors that contribute to negative changes to gene expression are unhealthy diet and lifestyle, nutrient deficiencies, toxins, and stress, to name a few. The good news is that you can alter your genetic expression and refine your genes to optimize your health and your life.

Single Nucleotide Polymorphisms (SNPs)

One of the hottest topics in genetics right now is a piece of the genetic puzzle that consists of genetic variations called SNPs (pronounced "snips"), which stands for single nucleotide polymorphisms. While many do not cause us issues, some can explain a lot about the behaviours, emotions, signs, and symptoms clients come to me with.

The most well-known SNP is the MTHFR gene, which can affect gene expression, DNA repair, and other cellular processes. A SNP in the MTHFR gene may result in increased risk of birth defects, miscarriages, infertility, irritability, cancer, and obsessiveness. In these cases, a small mutation in the SNP can have a huge effect.

Another well-studied SNP occurs in the COMT gene can lead to higher or lower levels of dopamine in the brain. This genetic variance determines how our body deals with stress as well has impacts cognitive or executive function. SNPs in COMT can result in irritability, memory changes, sleep issues, PMS, menopause symptoms, and workaholism.

Knowing Your Genetics is Important

The best part about knowing your genetics is you can be empowered to take charge of your health. Once you know your genetic tendencies, you can support your body and brain with diet and lifestyle that will allow you to reach your genetic potential.

Every moment of every day, your genes are spitting out instructions like the directions in a cookbook. They can give you a recipe for a delicious dessert, or a mistake or two can lead to a disgusting mess. The key is your genes are always coding and producing instructions. The choices you make every day can produce radically different outcomes.

For example, your genes can tell your gut lining to rebuild in a strong healthy way. Or, they can say, "Oh yeah, if you want to feed me all this junk and bombard me with things to do, I'll show you by creating a weak, leaky gut. Have fun with weight gain, fatigue, nutrient deficiencies, and immune issues." The same happens for our skin. If you're not treating your body right, your genes will start to send the signal that you want dull, acne-prone skin and premature wrinkling.

Now, on the other hand, you can support your body's ability to regain health and you will be glowing in no time. Just like the wrong signals to your genes can make your cells, organs, and body perform sub-optimally, if you send the right signals, you'll experience incredible health.

Lastly, if you want to be forgetful, irritable, and suffer from addictions, anxiety, depression, and brain fog, then just give your brain the wrong instructions involving neurotransmitters that govern your thoughts, mood and emotions.

So, what negatively affects genes, and what can you do to support your health by helping your body to express the right genes? Here are a few things that can cause the expression of harmful genes:

- Sugar
- Insufficient protein (big problem in my patient population)
- Not enough healthy fat
- Too much processed food
- Too many carbs
- A shortage of key nutrients
- Sedentary lifestyle or over-exercising
- Electrolyte deficiency and dehydration
- Stress
- Free radicals (oxidative stress)
- Not enough sleep
- Inconsistent sleep patterns
- Altered circadian rhythm
- Toxins in water, air, food, cleaning and personal care products
- Chronic stress
- Chronic underlying infections

- Chronic inflammation

What is Methylation?

There is a famous study in twin mice where researchers studied why and how two genetically identical mice could look completely different. In the study, both mice had DNA with a strong genetic potential for obesity, cardiovascular disease, and cancer, but only one of them was actually unhealthy. The mystery was solved by the concept of methylation, the ability to manipulate genes to create health rather than disease and illness. By methylating certain genes, you can turn off your genetic tendency for obesity and even disease!

Methylation comes into play with weight gain by helping to create a key compound called carnitine, which helps your body burn fat for fuel. When you're burning fat for fuel, your blood sugars are stable. Spikes and dips in blood sugar leads to anxiety, insulin resistance, overeating, and cravings for carbohydrates in an effort to boost energy and create stability. In addition, when your body is able to convert fat into energy to be utilized, you have energy, you can maintain a healthy weight, and cravings are under control.

Why You are Not Methylating Properly

Here are the top reasons why your genes may not be properly methylated:

You're not consuming real food — If you do nothing else, make sure to eat a whole-food, plant-based diet. If it comes from the ground and has a mother then go for it (preferably organic and hormone-free). If you are deficient in key vitamins, nutrients, and protein, your genes will not methylate properly.

You are consuming folic acid — Let's set the record straight on this one. The natural form of vitamin B6 is called folate. The active version of folate is called methylfolate because it is methylated and ready for the body to use. If you have issues with methylation, you want to consume lots of folate, which you can get from dark leafy greens. The synthetic form of B6 is called folic acid. It is found in processed foods and unfortunately in our grains (bread, cereal, cornmeal, flour, pasta, rice, other grains) and many poor-quality prenatal vitamins. To be clear, vitamin B6 is very important during pregnancy, but I would recommend the activated methylfolate over synthetic folic acid because the synthetic form is not useful for the body until it is activated.

To create more chaos, folic acid binds to receptors on your cells and blocks natural folate from binding. Even if you are consuming foods like leafy green vegetables and you think you are getting enough folate, it will likely be struggling to get into cells because the receptors are blocked. Without enough methylfolate you risk methylation deficiencies. In short, synthetic folic acid blocks methylation. If you are looking to supplement with folate, choose methylfolate. If the bottle says folic acid, throw it away.

In addition, if you have known methylation issues, I would highly recommend a paleo-style diet. That will remove the grains mentioned above, which are "enriched" with folic acid.

You are not sleeping properly — Aim to start winding down for bed at 9 pm. Journal, have a bath with Epsom salts, or meditate with lavender essential oil. This will bring you into a parasympathetic state to allow you to get to bed by 10 pm. Get at least eight hours of sleep per night, because if you don't, you risk not methylating adequately. Methylation is required for melatonin production, a hormone that helps you fall asleep and stay asleep. Choosing to lose out on sleep will create a vicious cycle, so stop it now.

You are stressed out — When you're stressed, methyl groups are added at a much higher rate than when you are in a calm and relaxed state. In order to keep up with the demand, you will require more methyl donors. But, if you're not consuming the right foods that contain the right macronutrients, you will be in trouble.

You are in toxic overload — Your liver's natural detoxification mechanisms rely on glutathione, which requires methylation. If you have poor methylation, you will have poor detoxification. In this world where we are calling upon our natural detox defenses at an overwhelming rate, our methyl donors frantically try to keep up and often fail.

You exercise too much or too little — I am the biggest fan of exercise, and I recommend all my patients engage in physical activity every day, no exceptions. But, doing too much or the wrong types of exercise can negatively affect methylation. While the right exercise in the right amount at the right intensity can create new patterns of methylation, too much exercise can be a stress on the body. Combined with an inadequate diet, that stress can leave you vulnerable.

Does This Sound Like You?

Every day, your genes are telling your metabolism to run fast or slow, to have energy or not, to lose weight or gain weight. They also provide instructions to your brain that affect mood and mental focus, helping to determine whether you feel anxious or calm, depressed or optimistic, focused or scattered.

Your genes are very complex and they always writing various codes and instructions. Focusing on one gene is only one small part of the conversation. You really need to look at all the genes as a whole, which is why I recommend genetic testing for you and your family. But, in this section we are going to zero in on three key genes that affect your energy, mood, and waistline. And, these three genes are all affected by methylation.

Choline — The production of phosphatidylcholine from choline involves methylation. Phosphatidylcholine is a key element of cell membranes. Phosphatidylcholine also plays a role in new cell formation, as well as the production of bile. If you do not have adequate bile, you are at an increased risk for unhealthy bacteria growing in the small intestine, and developing a condition called SIBO or small intestine bacterial overgrowth (bacteria should not be in the small intestine). Food sources of choline I recommend are eggs, fish, meats and nuts. In addition, you can consider supplementing but ensure your choline is not sourced from soy.

Creatine — Creatine also requires methylation. Glycocyamine, a metabolite of the amino acid glycine, is methylated to produce creatine. Creatine is important for energy production, as well as muscle function and brain health. In order to produce adequate creatine, you of course need glycine. Food sources of glycine I recommend are eggs, fish, and meats.

Melatonin — This master sleep hormone is produced when serotonin is methylated. Serotonin is an important chemical and neurotransmitter in the human body. It is believed to help regulate mood and social behaviour, appetite and digestion, sleep, memory, and sexual desire and function. When serotonin production is low, melatonin is affected. When methylation is impaired, melatonin is also affected.

How Methylation is Related to Detoxification

Right now, MTHFR is all the hype and for good reason. It kicks off the methylation cycle. Hundreds of reactions in your body rely on methylation, everything from digestion, mood, cellular regeneration, and detoxification. All these processes require methyl groups.

To understand the methylation cycle, think of a row of dominos all lined up. As the first domino starts to fall, each domino will start toppling the next. If one domino is out of line or gets jammed, the rest of the process cannot work.

MTHFR is the ball or force that starts the domino cascade, and then the methyl group is passed along during the methylation cycle. At the end of the methyl passing game is SAMe (S-adenosylmethionine). SAMe ultimately passes the methyl group onto all the critical processes in the body. After SAMe passes on the methyl group, it become homocysteine, the end product of methylation. To complete the cycle, if all is well, homocysteine goes back into the methylation cycle and the process starts all over. This entire process does require key nutrients like B6, B12 and folate to operate smoothly.

If you are under stress (physical, mental, or emotional) and have a lot of toxins, free radicals, inflammation, and oxidative stress in your body, then homocysteine is redirected to make glutathione, a key detox element. Now your homocysteine is pulled out of the methylation cycle to clean up the immediate mess, and the rest of the processes that require methylation get placed on the backburner. This is when symptoms arise.

Send Your Liver Some Lovin'

Want yet another reason to love your liver? (Go back and read Chapter 2 if you skipped over it. You'll learn why your liver is so incredibly important.) Well, in addition to detoxification, 85% of methylation occurs in the liver. So, you want to support the liver as much as possible.

Also, remember how detoxification is important to ensure estrogen levels don't get out of control? Excess estrogen in women can lead to issues with PMS, menstruation, menopause, ovarian cancer, and breast cancer. To clear harmful chemicals and hormones, you need to be methylating properly. And, methylation is necessary to produce glutathione, the master antioxidant. Lack of glutathione means lack of detoxification.

So, what can you do to support your liver and help methylation in its cells?

- Avoid or reduce alcohol intake, especially if you have methylation deficits.
- Reduce your daily exposure to chemicals in your environment, as well as heavy metals.
- Support your body with key nutrients that correct nutrient deficiencies as well as promote detoxification.

- Avoid unnecessary medications that place an additional burden on the liver.

Additional Conditions Rooted in Methylation

Allergies — Histamine is the chemical mediator that is involved in allergies. It is a byproduct of the immune system, and levels need to be managed just right. Too much histamine produces the common allergy symptoms we see, and can even contribute to insomnia. Histamine requires methylation to be expelled, and impaired methylation may be an aggravating factor in allergy sufferers.

Heavy Metal Toxicity — Glutathione is the detox superhero that removes heavy metals like arsenic, but arsenic first must be inactivated by methylation. Sources of arsenic include air, processed foods, rice, and drinking water.

Estrogen Dominance — Estrogen is a "goldilocks" hormone that requires levels to be "just right." Estrogen dominance is very common due to environmental sources of estrogen. Estrogen dominance can lead to cellulite, heavy periods, endometriosis, fibrocystic breasts, PMS, menstrual issues, and increased risk of estrogen-related cancers. Because of this, it is really important that we support detoxification of estrogen. Methylation protects us from estrogen dominance because methylated estrogen is inactive.

How to Test Your Genes

An inexpensive way to test your genetics would be through www.23andme.com, but you will require additional software such as Ben Lynch's' Stratagene and a trained practitioner to help you interpret the raw data. Another option would be to order tests through https://youtrients.me.

Are Your Genes Causing Carb Cravings?

While reviewing all the common genetic SNPs would be a novel in itself, I wanted to highlight the MAOA gene because it is one that I often see in clients with mood swings and carb cravings. I personally also have the fast MAOA profile.

People who have fast MAOA crave carbs like they are the only food on the planet. For me, despite knowing better, being prepared with protein and fat-rich meals and trying every appetite suppressant I could not resist carbohydrates, especially at night. After consuming the carbohydrate-rich food (chocolate and crepes were my go-to's), I would feel amazing, but then I'd be flooded with guilt and felt like the weakest person on the planet. I started to think something was seriously wrong with me until I investigated my genetics. Knowing that I have the fast MAOA profile allowed me to recognize my body was just craving what it needed.

Here is why: the MAOA gene causes your body to process serotonin quickly. Serotonin is calm, happy, positive, self-confident the neurotransmitter. When serotonin levels are too low, you may feel depressed, second guess your abilities, have sleep disturbances, and have low libido. When your body eats through serotonin quickly, its only defense mechanism is to raise levels quickly again, and to do so we crave sugary, starchy foods. While protein contains tryptophan, carbohydrate-rich foods contain tryptophan that can absorbed at a much faster rate.[63]

Recall from Chapter 7 that serotonin is methylated to form melatonin. So, if you have fast MAOA and you eat through serotonin quickly, you may find yourself waking yourself up in the middle of the night. This is because if you break down serotonin too fast, your levels of melatonin will be low.

---

[63] Spadaro, Paola A., et al. "A refined high carbohydrate diet is associated with changes in the serotonin pathway and visceral obesity." Genetics research 97 (2015).

The secret sauce is not necessarily to supplement with 5-HTP (precursor to serotonin) or melatonin, although these may be helpful. Instead, you should consume adequate levels of protein throughout the day. In doing so, neurotransmitter levels will be more stable. Recall carbohydrate-rich foods, especially simple carbohydrates, will result in a much greater spike in serotonin, followed by a rapid decline. The goal is sustained, balanced levels, so focus on eating complex carbohydrates and protein throughout the day.

By doing this, you will experience fewer food cravings and mood swings, better sleep cycles, and thus you will be less likely to fall victim to binging. Spinach, seaweed, mushrooms, pumpkin seeds, turnip greens, asparagus, and meat proteins are all great options because they contain tryptophan, a nutrient required to produce serotonin.

The other important piece is to manage stress. If stress is a factor that increases your carb cravings as it does for me, it is your responsibility to recognize when you are pushing yourself too hard and find ways to bring your stress level down by taking a break and going for a walk or doing five to ten minutes of meditation.

How to Promote Healthy Genes

In summary, here are the seven things you should add to your routine and lifestyle to help promote healthy gene expression and methylation:

- Sleep
- Remove toxicity
- Manage stress
- Eat lots of dark leafy greens
- Eat protein
- Drink clean water
- Supplement smartly

CHAPTER TWELVE

Sleep

Even with the very best nutrition and exercise routine, if your sleep is off, there is work to be done. Here's why sleep is so important to your waistline, energy, and libido.

Sleep and Weight Gain

The more of the hormone ghrelin you produce, the more you stimulate hunger while also reducing the number of calories you burn (your metabolism) and increasing the amount fat you store. In other words, you need to control leptin and ghrelin to successfully lose weight, but sleep deprivation makes that nearly impossible. (Refer back to Chapter 6 for a detailed review of the fat hormones.)

In fact, one 2004 study showed that participants with short sleep (five hours per night) had reduced leptin and elevated ghrelin compared to those who got more sleep (eight hours per night). These differences in leptin and ghrelin are likely to increase appetite, possibly explaining the increased BMI observed with short sleep duration.[64]

Sleep and Libido

I consider sex drive as a key indicator of overall physical and mental health, yet sadly, the state of women's health, longevity, and happiness is declining. As a result, low libido is common, and in most cases, the root cause is hormonal. The truth is hormones matter and how they interact can make or break sexual interest, and even toe-curling orgasms. Let's face it: If you'd rather scroll through Facebook than have sex, there's a good chance there's a hormone problem.

In many regards, sexuality can be viewed as a portal to other areas of your life. When you optimize your sex life, there are many resulting benefits you may not even realize. You may even begin to find freedom in other aspects of your life where there was once struggle whether you were conscious of it before or not. You heal from the inside out, which is far better and more sustainable than seeking the latest band-aid to the problem. This is true no matter how often you have sex and what sexuality looks like for you.

After working with hundreds of people who want to get their mojo back, I know how important sleep is to a healthy sex drive.

Key hormones such as progesterone and testosterone, which play a significant role in libido, are negatively impacted by lack of sleep. Reports of decreased testosterone following one night of total sleep deprivation have varied from 18.5% to 30.4% decreases in plasma testosterone.[65,66] One study also reported that one night of sleep

---

[64] Taheri, Shahrad, et al. "Short sleep duration is associated with reduced leptin, elevated ghrelin, and increased body mass index." *PLoS medicine* 1.3 (2004): e62.

[65] Cortes-Gallegos, V., et al. "Sleep deprivation reduces circulating androgens in healthy men." *Archives of andrology* 10.1 (1983): 33-37.

[66] Gonzalez-Santos, M. R., et al. "Sleep deprivation and adaptive hormonal

deprivation reduced progesterone but not estradiol in women.[67] Additionally, in female nurses working night shifts, 53% of women studied experienced alterations in their typical menstrual cycles.[68] Thus, it is very possible that just one night of sleep restriction can have profound effects on sex hormones and libido.

Sleep and Mood

You probably have firsthand experience confirming that lack of sleep affects mood. After just one sleepless night, you may be more irritable, short-tempered, and vulnerable to stress. Once you sleep well, your mood returns to normal that is if sleep deprivation does not become chronic like it is for so many of my clients.

Studies have confirmed that even slight sleep deprivation has a significant effect on mood. Researchers from the University of Pennsylvania found that subjects who reduced their natural sleep duration by 33% for just one week reported feeling more stressed, angry, sad, foggy, and mentally exhausted. When the subjects resumed normal sleep, they reported a dramatic improvement in mood.[69]

One way sleep negatively impacts mood is through altering sex hormones. As discussed above, lack of sleep can reduce progesterone levels and changes in progesterone levels can alter one's mood and sense of well-being. This is because allopregnanolone, the progesterone metabolite, is a GABA-A receptor agonist. This means

---

responses of healthy men." *Archives of andrology* 22.3 (1989): 203-207.

[67] Carter, Jason R., et al. "Sympathetic neural responses to 24-hour sleep deprivation in humans: sex differences." *American Journal of Physiology-Heart and Circulatory Physiology* 302.10 (2012): H1991-H1997.

[68] Labyak, Susan, et al. "Effects of shiftwork on sleep and menstrual function in nurses." *Health care for women international* 23.6-7 (2002): 703-714.

[69] Dinges, David F., et al. "Cumulative sleepiness, mood disturbance, and psychomotor vigilance performance decrements during a week of sleep restricted to 4–5 hours per night." *Sleep* 20.4 (1997): 267-277.

that allopregnanolone binds to GABA-A receptors.[70] Thus, with lower progesterone levels, GABA function decreases. As the main inhibitory neurotransmitter, GABA plays roles in promoting calmness, good mood, and sleep.[71]

How to Improve Your Sleep

Here are a few simple strategies to help optimize your sleep:

- Avoid blue light exposure one hour before bedtime. Avoid all electronics and wear blue blocking glasses.
- Read a book in the evening while wearing blue light blocking glasses under dim lighting such as a salt lamp.
- Have a bath with 1-2 cups of Epsom salts. Epson salts provide a dose of magnesium that can be absorbed through the skin.
- Do not consume caffeine late in the day.
- Avoid stimulating activities such as exercise before bed.
- Sleep in a cold, dark room.
- Consume magnesium threonate or magnesium bisglycinate during the day as well as a larger dose before bed.
- Drink sleepy time tea (chamomile, passion flower, valerian)
- Consider supplementing with 1-10mg of melatonin (liposomal is best) 30 minutes to 1 hour before bed.

---

[70] Follesa, Paolo, et al. "Allopregnanolone synthesis in cerebellar granule cells: roles in regulation of GABAA receptor expression and function during progesterone treatment and withdrawal." *Molecular Pharmacology* 57.6 (2000): 1262-1270.

[71] Ehlen, J. Christopher, et al. "GABA involvement in the circadian regulation of sleep." *GABA and Sleep*. Springer, Basel, 2010. 303-321.

CHAPTER THIRTEEN

Nutrition

I AM SO PASSIONATE ABOUT INDIVIDUALIZED CARE AND BELIEVE THERE IS NO "**ONE**-SIZE-FITS-ALL" APPROACH TO NUTRITION. With this being said, I do believe that my Wild Side Wellness is the ideal plan to master the general foundations of health.

If you are a busy woman with incredibly important roles to fill, a wife, mother, business owner, entrepreneur, or leader, then you know how debilitating it can be when you do not feel your best.

I want you to feel like you are operating at 100% because your family, friends, community, and YOU deserve it.

I know what it feels like to be up and down with your fitness and nutrition. You have tried intense, stressful, quick fixes and while you see results, you feel depleted, overwhelmed and out of control.

You need a solution that helps you feel in control again. You want physical results – to look fit and toned – but are also looking to reset your metabolism, improve your energy, balance your hormones, and to burn fat more effectively.

You feel like you know what foods are "healthy" and which are not, but need a simplified and structured plan with support and accountability at every step.

How to Choose a Diet that Works for You

Consider Your Food Preferences — You'll never be likely to make a diet work if you don't integrate at least some of your favourite foods. This means if you prefer pasta and carbs over meat and vegetables, you might want to consider the Mediterranean diet. If you prefer rich foods that are high in fat, you should try the ketogenic diet. Making the right choice for you could make the difference between success and failure within the weight loss process.

Commit to Meal Planning — You're unlikely to stick to your diet if you're constantly rushing and don't have time to carefully consider your meal options. This means it's important to dedicate some time during the week to meal planning. Just a few minutes a week can help you determine how best to stick to your healthy eating habits. You should review your options at the grocery store and plan for meals that include only the healthiest foods.

Track Your Progress — While you shouldn't be checking your weight on a daily basis, you should have a way of measuring weight loss progress. You might consider a weekly chart that gives you all the information on your diet and your weight as time passes. This will help motivate you to continue your diet as you see your results improve.

What is Intermittent Fasting?

In my opinion, intermittent fasting is the number one under-utilized health tool. In North America we have been conditioned to eat as soon as our eyes open in the morning and many folks snack right up until when they hit the sack. Fasting is most known for its use in fat loss, but it offers so much more than lost inches.

Before we go into the science of fasting and fat burning, you must understand the difference between the "fed" state and the "fasted" state. Your body is in a fed state when it is digesting and absorbing food. It starts when you begin eating and lasts anywhere from three to five hours as your body digests, breaks down, and absorbs food. It is hard for the body to burn fat in a fed state because insulin levels are elevated.

After digestion and absorption, your body goes into the post-absorptive state, which means you are no longer processing food. This state lasts 8-12 hours after your last meal, at which point you are in a fasted state. In the fasted state, insulin levels are low and the body is able to use fat as a fuel source. However, most people do not leave 12 hours between meals, and therefore never achieve a fasted state. This is why people who practice intermittent fasting will lose body fat without changing what they eat or how much they eat. The fasted state puts your body into a fat-burning mode that you cannot achieve while eating five to six times per day.

There is a lot of initial evidence to suggest that temporary periodic fasting can induce long lasting changes that can be beneficial against aging and chronic disease.

Even if you took a cocktail of drugs, very potent ones, you will never get close to what fasting does! Let's go over my favourite benefits of intermittent fasting.

Benefit #1: Fasting and Longevity

Many studies have shown that fasted mice live longer, and unlike caloric restricted mice, the fasted mice were not physically stunted.[72]

---

[72] Honjoh, Sakiko, et al. "Signalling through RHEB-1 mediates intermittent

In these studies, mice that fast also had fewer signs of cancer, heart disease, and neurodegeneration. Fasting increases one's lifespan, but more importantly, it increases one's "health span." Health span is the amount of time you live without chronic age-related diseases. The possible mechanism by which fasting increases health span is that when you fast, your body reduces the amount of IGF-1 it makes. Lower amounts of circulating levels of IGF-1 may play a role in reducing your risk of diseases of aging because it switches on a number of repair genes.[73]

Benefit #2: Fasting and Autophagy

One of the changes noted during fasting is that the body switches on a process called "autophagy." Autophagy literally means to "self-eat." It is a process by which the body breaks down and recycles old and tired cells. Just like we must take our cars in for repairs and tune ups, it is important to get rid of damaged or aging cells in our bodies. Fasting acts as the spring clean, getting rid of the old and allowing opportunity for new cells (which behave properly) to proliferate.[74,75,76,77]

fasting-induced longevity in *C. elegans.*" *Nature* 457.7230 (2009): 726-730.

[73] Cheng, Chia-Wei, et al. "Prolonged fasting reduces IGF-1/PKA to promote hematopoietic-stem-cell-based regeneration and reverse immunosuppression." *Cell stem cell* 14.6 (2014): 810-823.

[74] Madeo, Frank, Nektarios Tavernarakis, and Guido Kroemer. "Can autophagy promote longevity?." *Nature cell biology* 12.9 (2010): 842-846.

[75] Mammucari, Cristina, et al. "FoxO3 controls autophagy in skeletal muscle in vivo." *Cell metabolism* 6.6 (2007): 458-471.

[76] Alirezaei, Mehrdad, et al. "Short-term fasting induces profound neuronal autophagy." *Autophagy* 6.6 (2010): 702-710.

[77] Vanhorebeek, Ilse, et al. "Insufficient activation of autophagy allows cellular damage to accumulate in critically ill patients." *The Journal of Clinical Endocrinology & Metabolism* 96.4 (2011): E633-E645.

Benefit #3: Fasting and Stem Cell Regeneration

When we fast, our bodies want to save energy. One of the ways our bodies converse energy is by recycling immune cells that are not needed, especially those which are damaged. The body can use the components of these cells for fuel. Yes, white blood cells have been shown to decrease with prolonged fasting (making you more prone to infection), but a short fast results in a rebound effect with the creation of new, more active cells.[78]

Fasting also has the ability to impact our genetics. One interesting area of research is that fasting appears to be able to reduce the activity of the PKA gene. This gene encodes or provides the blueprint to produce an enzyme that would normally reduce regeneration. Thus, when the PKA gene expression is reduced, the enzyme is not generated and stem cells can start proliferating. What is really cool is the potential impact this has on the aging process. The researchers who published these findings have hypothesized that if your immune system is not as effective as it was (either due to age or chemotherapy) then intermittent fasting (and the changes it causes to genetics) may help regenerate it.[79]

Benefit #4: Fasting is NOT Just Caloric Restriction

There is a misconception out there that fasting results in weight loss because it is merely a calorie deficit, but I believe it is much more.

Research out of Salk Institute for Biological Studies looked at two groups of mice.[80] Both groups were fed the exact same high-fat diet.

---

[78] Cheng, Chia-Wei, et al. "Prolonged fasting reduces IGF-1/PKA to promote hematopoietic-stem-cell-based regeneration and reverse immunosuppression." *Cell stem cell* 14.6 (2014): 810-823.

[79] Cheng, Chia-Wei, et al. "Prolonged fasting reduces IGF-1/PKA to promote hematopoietic-stem-cell-based regeneration and reverse immunosuppression." *Cell stem cell* 14.6 (2014): 810-823.

[80] Chaix, Amandine, et al. "Time-restricted feeding is a preventative and

Group 1 was allowed to eat whenever they wanted (ad libitum), whereas Group 2 had to eat within an eight-hour feeding window (Time Restricted Feeding or TRF).

After 100 days, the group that was allowed to eat all day developed high cholesterol, high blood glucose, and liver damage. In contrast, the intermittent fasting group gained 28% less weight, suffered less liver damage, had lower levels of chronic inflammation. This suggests intermittent fasting may be able to reduce the risk of a number of diseases such as Alzheimer's disease, heart disease, cancer, and stroke.

WHY? How can this be?

One possible mechanism is that when you eat, your insulin levels are elevated and your body is stuck in storage mode. The rats that were always nibbling, so they always had high insulin, resulting in obesity and liver damage.

Benefit #5: Fasting and Diabetes

Let's review a key hormone when it comes insulin resistance and diabetes.

Insulin is a hormone that is similar to IGF-1 that we talked about above. It tends to increase cell turnover and reduce autophagy (clearing of old cells). Aside from this, insulin is best known for its role in regulating blood sugar.

When we eat foods, particularly carbohydrates, our blood sugar levels rise and our pancreas starts to pump out insulin in response. Glucose is typically the primary fuel source for energy, BUT high circulating levels of glucose are toxic. The primary role of insulin is to regulate blood glucose levels. We do not want blood sugar too high

---

therapeutic intervention against diverse nutritional challenges." *Cell metabolism* 20.6 (2014): 991-1005.

or too low! In order to do this, insulin extracts glucose from blood and sends it to the liver to be stored in the form of glycogen. Insulin is also a fat controller and inhibits lipolysis, the breakdown of stored body fat. And, at the same time it forces cells to take up and store fat from your body.

So, in summary, high levels of Insulin increases fat storage and low levels lead to depletion of fat stores.

Where we run into problems is if we frequently eat high-carbohydrate meals. Your pancreas copes to the best of its ability by pumping out more and more insulin. Eventually your cells will rebel and become resistant to the effect. It's kind of like when your kids are yelling, "MOM! MOM! MOM!" and eventually you can't help but tune them out.

Your cells too eventually stop responding to insulin, and your blood glucose stays permanently high. Now unfortunately for you, you've joined the 422 million people around the world who have type 2 diabetes. This mind-blowing statistic is up from 108 million people living with type 2 diabetes in 1980.[81]

Type 2 diabetes is a PREVENTABLE disease that you do not want to suffer with. According to the World Health Organization, "Diabetes can be treated and its consequences avoided or delayed with diet, physical activity, medication, and regular screening and treatment for complications." Diabetes is associated with increased risk of dementia, brain shrinkage, amputation, heart attack, kidney disease, and blindness. The good news is a 2005 study showed that in just two weeks of intermittent fasting, you can positively impact your body's ability to respond to insulin.[82]

---

[81] http://www.who.int/mediacentre/factsheets/fs312/en/

[82] N. Halberg, M. Henricksen, N. Söderhamn, B. Stallknecht, T. Ploug, P. Scherling, and F. Dela, Department of Muscle Research Centre, The Panum Institute, University of Copenhagen, Denmark, "Effect of intermittent fasting and refeeding on insulin action in healthy men," *Journal of Applied Physiology* (December 2005): 2128-36.

Fasting is so powerful because it provides a rest for your pancreas, which will boost the effectiveness of the insulin it produces in response to elevated blood glucose. Increased insulin sensitivity will reduce your risk of obesity, diabetes, heart disease, and cognitive decline.

Carb Cycling

You have probably been hearing more and more about carb cycling, and for good reason! This is a superior, upper level nutrition plan that allows for variety and flexibility in your diet. Essentially carb cycling mixes higher carbohydrate days with lower carbohydrate days with the goal of achieving fat loss.

Overall, the number of calories you consume in one week stays consistent, but what changes is your macronutrients or "macros." Typically, there are some low carb days, regular carb days and high carb days. Doing this allows for "discretionary" calories, which translates to consuming foods you crave (within reason) without suffering as many of the negative consequences that a purely low carb plan would have.

Why Carb Cycling is Important

Consuming a diet low in carbohydrates depletes glycogen levels and forces your body to break down fat and use ketones for fuel. This is what you want to happen if you are looking to lose fat. The issue is if you consume a low carb diet every single day, you may have a marked reduction in your physical performance. By incorporating higher carbohydrate days, you are able to refuel your muscles so that your strength and endurance are not compromised.

Another negative aspect of a strict low carbohydrate diet is lack of flexibility, cravings, difficulty focusing, and a reduction in metabolic rate (your metabolism). Cycling your carbs, as well as adding exercise to your plan, will help to offset these factors. Carb cycling can help you lose stubborn fat, but before you jump in, here are some things you need to know.

You Need a Strategic Plan

Entering into a program like this without a game plan of how you intend to combine your diet and exercise will not result in the outcome you hoped for. One of the very first things you need to do is to schedule your highest carb days on the days when you lift heavy weights or do your hardest workout. In my program, we combine high carb days with leg days or a full-body workout in order to provide the fuel to get through these killer workouts. This allows you to lift heavier, become stronger, and it aids in the recovery process.

One thing to keep in mind is that this type of lifestyle will require more planning initially until you get comfortable with the process. To make things foolproof I suggest my clients track their macros and caloric intake. Spending one day planning out your week's meals will also help to keep you on track.

Keep Your Target Weekly Caloric Intake Consistent

Before starting a carb cycling program, you must calculate your total weekly caloric intake. Your caloric intake should be based off your age, height, weight, fitness level, and goals. This value must remain fairly consistent on a weekly basis to achieve overall fat loss. Keep in mind an overall caloric deficit is required for weight loss, but it not the only component. For sustainable fat loss that doesn't negatively impact your hormones or metabolism, carb cycling is key.

Feeling "Puffy" After High Carb Days is Normal

When you load up on carbohydrates, water will also be pulled into your muscles, so expect to feel like you have gained some water weight. When carbohydrates are consumed, your body will convert them into glycogen that is then stored in your muscles. Your body is constantly trying to maintain balance or "homeostasis." When you eat carbs, your kidneys are signaled to retain more sodium. For every gram of glycogen, 2.7 grams of water is stored in order to maintain sodium-blood concentration. Typically, clients describe themselves as feeling "puffy." If you are already lean you will likely notice this the next day, but don't be alarmed. It will recede when you return to your regular or low carbohydrate days.

Low Carb Days Are Not Always Pretty

If your body is used to consuming a high carbohydrate diet or one that is rich in "unhealthy foods," there is going to be an adjustment phase. Your body is used to burning glucose for energy, but now it needs to transition into ketosis and use fats (ketones) for fuel. For some, this period brings forth some unpleasant symptoms. Often described as the "Ketosis Flu," some report experiencing headaches, nausea, brain fog, skin rash, and/or fatigue. To prevent these feelings, drink plenty of water, be sure to consume your fats, and maintain your electrolytes. Like any new lifestyle change, it takes weeks to form a habit, so stick with it.

High Carbohydrate Does Not Mean a Feeding Frenzy

If your goal is fat loss, you cannot expect to achieve the results you want if you overdo it on high carb days. Stay away from high fructose corn syrup and white sugar. While a treat is absolutely okay every once in a while, the goal should be to consume foods that will provide dense nutrition. If you use up your carbohydrates on simple sugars, there is a greater chance that this glucose will be converted and stored as fat. My advice is to choose complex carbohydrates such as quinoa, sweet potatoes, brown rice, starchy vegetables, and so on. To maximize your results further, focus on root vegetables for your carb sources and maintain a paleo diet.

Lower Fat on High Carbohydrate Days

In order to achieve an overall weekly caloric deficit, on high carbohydrate days it will be necessary to reduce your dietary fat intake. Remember that it's very important to keep your weekly calories consistent. Another option would be to offset the additional calories consumed on a high-carb day with a low-calorie day. Incorporating intermittent fasting is a strategy to help you achieve this.

I hope you have found this information useful and are now empowered with confidence to get started with carb cycling. I believe carb cycling when combined with intermittent fasting and a strategic exercise plan is a superior lifestyle for those who wish to maintain workout performance and lean muscle mass. In my opinion, this is a key way to prevent plateaus and lose fat.

How to Properly Fuel for Fat Loss

"What should I eat after a workout?" This is a topic that frequently gets discussed in my online programs. There is no one-size-fits-all approach, but I'd like to share with you what I have personally have found to be most effective.

You've probably heard the saying, "timing is everything," and properly refuelling after a workout is no exception. Eating the right foods at the right time for the right reason is crucial to replenishing your body's energy stores and prepping you for your next workout. There is no one-size-fits-all approach to refuelling recommendations. In fact, when it comes to refuelling, you have a variety of different options. What is recommended will change depending on your goals and the type of workouts you are engaging in.

Here is what I personally have found to maximize the effectiveness of my workouts. Specifically, I follow a carb cycling and intermittent fasting nutrition plan, and I build my exercise plan around it.

Below you will find an outline of what to eat after your workouts.

You will learn how I refuel my body following a cardio sprint workout vs a heavy weight training session. Keep in mind my goals are fat loss while maintaining/gaining lean muscle mass.

What to Eat After Cardio Sprint Days

Every day, I skip breakfast. I fast until at least noon. In the morning I am consuming water and black coffee, and I supplement with branch chain amino acids (BCAAs) and probiotics. On low carb days you may also want to add in exogenous keytones to maintain mental clarity, energy, and focus.

Twice a week, I do sprint training follow by low-intensity cardio. Sprint training depletes glycogen stores so my body can make a faster switch to burning triglycerides (or fat) for fuel. The low-intensity cardio further promotes fat breakdown. Typically, I try to do my sprints in the morning and I do them fasted. I then remain fasted for at least one to two hours after my sprints. To protect my muscles from being broken down and used for fuel, I consume BCAAs.

BCAAs — leucine, isoleucine and valine — are found in muscle proteins. During exercise, muscles are broken down. Research has shown BCAA supplementation before exercise improves muscle recovery by decreasing the release of essential amino acids from exercising muscle.[83] BCAA supplementation just prior to exercise also increases protein synthesis (muscle growth), reduces muscle soreness, and increases function.

What to Eat After Heavy Weight Days

I've been experimenting with doing my heavy weight (strength training) workout fasted. I will definitely consume BCAAs prior to a

---

[83] Jackman, Sarah R. et al. "Branched-Chain Amino Acid Ingestion Can Ameliorate Soreness From Eccentric Exercise". Medicine & Science in Sports & Exercise 42.5 (2010): 962-970. Web.

heavy weight workout, as well as a teaspoon of coconut oil in my coffee. I try to time my heavy weight workout closer to when I will be breaking my fast. If I am planning on breaking my fast at 1 o'clock, I aim to do my workout anywhere from 10 o'clock to 12 o'clock. I find I get hungry after a full-body workout and don't want to wait long to eat. You also don't want to wait too long to consume your protein and carbohydrates after a heavy weight workout because these macros help repair your muscles.

One concern I had about doing heavy weight workouts fasted is that I would not have as much strength. I have been doing fasted heavy weight workouts for months now and I have not noticed this being an issue.

One exception to this is LEG day. I always pair leg day with my high carb day. I like to consume some carbs prior to my leg workout to provide me the additional energy to max out my leg workout. The majority of my remaining carbs I like to consume following my leg workout. I still fast on leg day until at least noon.

What If You Have to Work out in the AM?

For my clients who only can work out first thing, I recommend trying both your cardio speed bursts and your heavy weight workouts fasted and see how you feel. Personally, I would highly recommend consuming BCAAs if this is your plan. If you find that you are hungry, you may need to break your fast early and have your last meal earlier. Try your best to stick to your intermittent fasting feeding window. You can also add coconut oil or MCT oil to black coffee to see if that is enough to regulate your blood sugars. If you absolutely feel like you need to consume something, I would suggest a low-carb protein shake immediately after your workout.

What If You Have to Work out in the PM?

If there is no way for you to work out in the morning, here is what I would suggest and do. I would do cardio workouts after your last meal. You will deplete your glycogen stores and switch to burning triglycerides until you break your fast the following day.

For your heavy weight workouts, I would do them at least 30 minutes to an hour away from food so you don't develop cramps and feel nauseous. Following your heavy weight workouts, consume the rest of your macros for the day.

The Bottom Line

Here's the deal: the best time to exercise is when you are ACTUALLY going to do it. Planning is everything. I see this time and time again. The clients who are most successful have a plan and they stick to it.

If you know you are NOT going to exercise after work, then find time to complete the workout in the morning or at lunch. While timing your food around your workouts may put you at a slight advantage, not doing your workout at all will definitely put you at a disadvantage.

It is also very important to listen to your body. If you feel nauseous, dizzy, or weak during your fasted workouts, then fasted training is probably not for you. If you feel your muscles are more sore post workout then normal, then consider taking a BCAA supplement around your workout, or consuming a protein shake at minimum sooner after your workout.

CHAPTER FOURTEEN

Workouts

"**T**HERE IS NO PILL THAT IS MORE EFFECTIVE AT REDUCING MORBIDITY AND MORTALITY AS EXERCISE."

There is an overwhelming amount of supportive evidence of the benefits of daily exercise. Exercise burns calories; in fact, high intensity interval training (HIIT) has been shown to burn extra calories for up to 72 hours! Exercise builds muscle, but stimulating muscle-building hormones means you will burn more calories at rest.

We know what exercise changes our hormones, and in turn our hormones can dictate the degree of results we see in the gym. For instance, exercise reduces hormones that interfere with our bodies' ability to release fat by cranking up PPARs (peroxisome proliferator-activated receptors), the regulators of fat metabolism and insulin sensitivity in our muscle cells. The right type of exercise has also been shown to positively influence cortisol as well as estrogen levels, which is great news for our adrenals.

Lastly, exercise has many positive changes on brain neurochemistry such increasing dopamine and endorphins, our natural painkillers, and increasing serotonin our happy hormone. Many of my clients report improved mental clarity and memory with exercise alone, as well as decreased episodes of anxiety and depression.

When done in the right amounts, at the right time, and for the right reasons, exercise can improve the balance of all energy-boosting fat loss hormones. Whether you decided to first focus on diet and lifestyle and incorporate exercise in a couple weeks, or start with exercise right away, it is a vital component to my Wild Side plan. As you begin to incorporate more movement and exercise, you will notice changes to your mental state and physical body. Action precedes motivation. Take action and you will see your waistline shrink and your self-image will improve. Exercise in my opinion has profound restorative powers and is one of the top things you can do to improve your overall health.

The Workout Split

For maximum energy and hormone balance, I recommend that you exercise five to six times per week. Each week I recommend you do three strength training days, two to three HIIT days and one yoga/walking day. I highly suggest you give your exercise priority in your day. This means have it scheduled firmly in your calendar. This will help you stick with your routine.

Why HIIT?

HIIT is a broad term for workouts that involve short periods of intense exercise alternated with recovery periods. One of the biggest advantages of HIIT is that you can get maximal health benefits in minimal time (10-30 minutes is all you need). In fact, researchers have found that HIIT burns up to 25–30% more calories than other forms of exercise.[84]

One of the ways HIIT helps you burn calories actually comes after you are done exercising. HIIT is also well known for its ability to ramp up your metabolic rate for hours after you work out.[85] HIIT also pushes your body to favour using fat for fuel rather than carbs. And, HIIT can get you amazing metabolic effects in a very short amount of time. In fact, one study from the University of Lethbridge in Canada showed that athletes get a similar metabolic boost from 30 minutes of running and just two minutes of sprint intervals (HIIT).[86]

My recommendation is to perform 10-20 minutes of HIIT training two to three times per week, followed up with 30 minutes of low intensity steady state (LISS) cardio.

Why Low Intensity Steady State cardio (LISS)?

In addition to HIIT, I ask my clients to engage in LISS cardio. The bottom line is that every step counts and walking keeps your heart rate in the fat burning mode. Walking curbs the negative effects of stress, can improve your sleep, and is ideal after a meal to balance blood sugar levels. One of my favourite studies on exercise showed that doing moderate intensity walking just 2-3 times per week can increase adiponectin by 260% and it remains elevated for 10 weeks.[87]

---

[84] Falcone, Paul H., et al. "Caloric expenditure of aerobic, resistance, or combined high-intensity interval training using a hydraulic resistance system in healthy men." *The Journal of Strength & Conditioning Research* 29.3 (2015): 779-785.

[85] Wingfield, Hailee L., et al. "The acute effect of exercise modality and nutrition manipulations on post-exercise resting energy expenditure and respiratory exchange ratio in women: a randomized trial." *Sports medicine-open* 1.1 (2015): 11.

[86] Hazell, Tom J., et al. "Two minutes of sprint-interval exercise elicits 24-hr oxygen consumption similar to that of 30 min of continuous endurance exercise." *International journal of sport nutrition and exercise metabolism* 22.4 (2012): 276-283.

[87] Kriketos, Adamandia D., et al. "Exercise increases adiponectin levels and

The increased adiponectin was seen after just one week which is amazing because it shows how fast our bodies can heal when given the correct stimulus.

Why Yoga?

Restorative yoga coupled with deep breathing is one of the best things you can do for HPA dysfunction. Yoga brings your body back into alignment, and focusing on your breath reduces stress and provides more oxygen to your cells. Regardless of your current fitness level, yoga can be adapted for you. Yoga not only offers fabulous benefits for calming your nervous system, restoring hormone balance but also strengthens your muscle and improves flexibility. A 2007 study out of Boston University School of Medicine showed that yoga can increase the calming neurotransmitter GABA and thus may be useful in the treatment of depression and anxiety.[88]

The benefits of yoga extend beyond subjective findings. Research shows that a yoga-based lifestyle intervention can effectively prevent and halt the progression of cardiovascular and metabolic disorders. The hypothesized mechanism of action of such benefit may be attributed to a reduction in weight and stress and improved sleep quality, as well as reduction in inflammation.[89]

Why Resistance or Strength Training?

Strength training is my ultimate favourite type of exercise due to the overwhelming body of evidence surrounding it. The effects of this

---

insulin sensitivity in humans." *Diabetes care* 27.2 (2004): 629-630.

[88] Streeter, Chris C., et al. "Yoga Asana sessions increase brain GABA levels: a pilot study." *The Journal of Alternative and Complementary Medicine* 13.4 (2007): 419-426.

[89] Sarvottam, Kumar, and Raj Kumar Yadav. "Obesity-related inflammation & cardiovascular disease: Efficacy of a yoga-based lifestyle intervention." The Indian journal of medical research 139.6 (2014): 822.

kind of exercise on metabolism, hormones, energy balance, and inflammatory markers is remarkable. Strength training improves muscle quality and improves insulin sensitivity throughout your entire body. It also reduces inflammation and increases adiponectin, a recipe for improved metabolic control and reduced risk of cardiovascular disease.

In terms of physiological math, the more muscle you have, the greater the number of calories you will burn at rest. Women from my Wild Side program who engage in specific resistance training will see significantly better results than those who only follow the diet.

Resistance training for weight loss also offers benefits over aerobic cardio training. This is because lactic acid builds up during resistance training. Research shows that high levels of blood lactic acid decrease blood pH levels, which then signal to the brain to release growth hormone.[90] The higher the growth hormone, the more intense your fat loss, so feel the burn!

Exercise Guidelines

Here are some general guidelines that I recommend you follow as you're putting together an exercise plan for weight loss:

1. Stay focused: When at the gym or working out from home, put away your phone and limit distractions. Set the intention at the start of your workout to be present.

2. Push to your max: In order to get maximum results from HIIT you must give 110% during the high intensity interval. Remember with weight training lactic acid build up is important so you should be experiencing near failure on your last rep.

3. Move with intention: With the Wild Side workouts you

---

[90] Godfrey, Richard J., et al. "The role of lactate in the exercise-induced human growth hormone response: evidence from McArdle disease." *British journal of sports medicine* 43.7 (2009): 521-525.

should be keeping your heart rate up as you move through the sets. The more you can keep your heart rate elevated, the more fat you will burn. Also, this helps to basically get your cardio and strength training workout done in one session. Benefits include better insulin control, increased growth hormone and elevated testosterone.

4. Aim for compound movements. A compound movement is simply one that works multiple muscle groups at once.

5. Choose short HIIT followed by 30 minutes of LISS. Doing this will maximize results with minimal time and effort. Walking provides the greatest results of boosting adiponectin when completed 2-3x per week at moderate intensity.

6. Calm down. Yoga is amazing for reducing stress and improving breathing. It also stimulates calming neurotransmitter release such as GABA.

7. Don't forget nutrient timing. It is important to properly fuel for your workouts to maximize fat loss. I recommend engaging in HIIT and LISS cardio in the fasted state. If possible, complete your HIIT/LISS cardio in the morning and maintain your fast until the afternoon. In terms of strength training, I recommend consuming a meal of carbohydrates and protein about an hour before a workout and again post workout, limiting fat post workout. This will encourage muscle gains and thus more fat loss in the future.

Strength Training: Choosing the Appropriate Weight

The weights you choose to use to complete the exercises needs to be challenging but not so much that your form is compromised. The last rep should be difficult. If you could do five more, the weight is not heavy enough. Time and time again, I see people who fail to get results because they do not lift weights to challenge their muscles. Your results and safety are my top priority, so consider hiring a personal trainer or join one of my programs if you need help getting started. Don't be afraid to get started; we are talking about an investment in your long-term health and wellbeing.

The Workout Schedule

Here is a workout schedule I recommend to many of my clients who want to get started with a basic strength training and exercise routine:

DAY	ACTIVITY
Monday	HIIT/LISS
Tuesday	Strength #1
Wednesday	HIIT/LISS
Thursday	Strength #2
Friday	Yoga, LISS optional
Saturday	Strength #3
Sunday	Rest/Yoga/LISS

To follow this plan, you should walk (40-60 minutes) 3-5 times per week (LISS), do a HIIT workout 2-3 times week, and strength train 3 times per week.

Easing Muscle Soreness

Delayed onset muscle soreness (DOMS) is the technical term for the aches and pains you feel after an intense workout. If you are just getting back into your exercise regime, this is a familiar experience.

The exact cause of muscle soreness is not known, but there are several hypothesized theories such as lactic acid buildup, muscle spasm, connective tissue damage, inflammation, and enzyme efflux. While one theory has yet to be proven, in my opinion, integration of two or more theories is the most likely explanation.

Delayed muscle soreness is an inconvenience for anyone working out, but for professional athletes it means a reduction in athletic performance. Another issue with DOMS is that the body naturally compensates for that soreness, resulting in unaccustomed stress on the ligaments and tendons, increasing the risk of injury.

Currently I am using my muscle tenderness as a motivation to keep going. For me, feeling "the burn" is a constant reminder that what I am doing is causing change. While some soreness is okay, I ensure it is not to a level that impacts my next workout or risks injury.

Lifestyle and supplemental therapies do exist to help alleviate the severity of muscle fatigue with evidence to support restoring maximal function ASAP and reducing the risk of injury.

If you're struggling with post-workout muscle soreness, these natural solutions may help your achy muscles get some relief:

Hydration — First and foremost! This is the most important thing you can do for your body. Loss of even a small percent of body weight through sweating can result in dehydration. Symptoms include fatigue, headaches, and diminished mental acuity. When rehydrating it is important to consider the amount of sodium lost through sweating. Adding in sodium to a replacement solution may be beneficial depending on the level of activity endured or how much you sweat. One study suggests 150% of fluid losses must be consumed to allow for complete fluid restoration.[91]

If water was not so critical to health, our bodies would not be made up of so much of it. If heat was not vitally important to survival, our bodies wouldn't spend so much energy maintaining a narrow thermic range.

Protein — Another basic principle of fitness is you need adequate protein in order to maintain muscle mass and function. Availability

---

[91] Burke, LM. "Nutrition For Post-Exercise Recovery.". Australian Journal of Science and Medicine in Sport 29.1 (1997): 3-10. Print.

of protein, particularly post-exercise, enhances muscle protein synthesis. In comparing athletes who consumed placebo (0 g carb, 0 g protein, 0 g fat), vs. control (8 g carb, 0 g protein, 3 g fat) vs. protein supplement (8 g carb, 10 g protein, 3 g fat), researchers found the protein group had fewer medical visits, less muscle soreness, and interestingly fewer infections. The authors concluded that consuming protein and carbohydrates post exercise will reduce muscle soreness And, protein consumption can be a therapeutic approach for the prevention of health problems in exercising populations.[92]

Contrast Showers — Contrast showers involve alternating hot and cold temperature application to cause alternating vasoconstriction and vasodilation. During contrast therapy, each alteration of temperature generally lasts for 30-120 seconds and is repeated two to five times. This treatment stimulates the metabolism of the tissues it is applied to. It stimulates circulation (increases oxygen absorption, increases CO_2 excretion), increases lactic acid removal, reduces inflammation and swelling, relieves stiffness and pain, and increases range of motion, all leading to a reduction in muscle fatigue and tension.[93]

Caffeine — For all of you coffee lovers out there like me, we are in luck. Finally, a study to support the addiction so many of us suffer with! Caffeine ingestion immediately before a resistance training not only enhances performance, but there are further beneficial effects of sustained caffeine ingestion in the days after the exercise! Days later, individuals in a 2013 study reported decreased soreness, which allowed the participants to increase the number of training sessions in a given time period.[94]

---

[92] Flakoll, P. J. "Postexercise Protein Supplementation Improves Health And Muscle Soreness During Basic Military Training In Marine Recruits". Journal of Applied Physiology 96.3 (2003): 951-956. Web.

[93] Wilcock, Ian M, John B Cronin, and Wayne A Hing. "Physiological Response To Water Immersion". Sports Medicine 36.9 (2006): 747-765. Web.

[94] Hurley, Caitlin F., Disa L. Hatfield, and Deborah Riebe. "The Effect Of Caffeine Ingestion On Delayed Onset Muscle Soreness". Journal of Strength and Conditioning Research (2013): 1. Web.

Magnesium — Suboptimal magnesium (Mg) levels are quite common in North Americans, and certain exercise appears to aggravate the consequences of this depletion.[95] In particular, exercise that promotes fatty acid mobilization, AKA lipolysis (long endurance type trainings), causes a decrease in plasma Mg.[96] Animal experiments show that Mg deficiency reduces physical performance and reduces the efficiency of energy metabolism, which can contribute to muscle soreness and recovery.[97] If physiological doses are administered for one month and positive effects are seen, this provides evidence that a deficiency may have existed.

Acupuncture — Competitive athletes are faced with the challenge of pushing their minds and bodies to the limit. When athletes consistently work at higher and higher intensities, their performance becomes hindered due to the accumulation of lactic acid in the muscles. Acupuncture is an effective strategy to reduce lactic acid levels so athletes can complete at their best, and it offers a faster, quicker recovery. Evidence from a 2011 study on elite basketball athletes showed acupuncture reduced HR_{max}, VO_2max, and blood lactic acid levels in athletes at 30 and 60 minutes post exercise.[98] The researchers concluded that acupuncture can enhance the recovery process after aggressive exercise. One possible explanation is that acupuncture increases circulation, which promotes flushing of lactic acid, thereby reducing recovery times for athletes.

Vitamin C — Traditionally, we've thought of vitamin C being used during colds and flus, but it turns out this antioxidant can do a lot more. Researchers led an investigation into whether or not vitamin

---

[95] Mooren, Frank C. et al. "Alterations Of Ionized Mg^{2+} In Human Blood After Exercise". Life Sciences 77.11 (2005): 1211-1225. Web.

[96] Rayssiguier, Y., et al. "Mg Water The Magnesium Web Site." *Magnesium Research* 3.2 (1990): 93-102.

[97] Navas, Francisco J. and Alfredo Córdova. "Effect Of Magnesium Supplementation And Training On Magnesium Tissue Distribution In Rats". Biological Trace Element Research 55.1-2 (1996): 213-213. Web.

[98] Lin, Zen-Pin, et al. "Effects of auricular acupuncture on heart rate, oxygen consumption and blood lactic acid for elite basketball athletes." *The American journal of Chinese medicine* 39.06 (2011): 1131-1138.

C supplementation before exercise could reduce muscle soreness proved effective.[99] This benefit is attributed to the antioxidant effects of vitamin C. As an antioxidant, it effectively reduces oxidation damage and reduces inflammation that occurs during exercise and contributes to muscle fatigue and post exercise soreness. If you are considering supplementing with vitamin C, talk to your doctor for a recommended dose. Consuming too much vitamin C may result in diarrhea.

Proteolytic Enzymes — The use of proteolytic enzymes in sport recovery is controversial. Although outdated, studies do exist that demonstrate administration of various proteolytic enzymes decreasing the amount of swelling and pain associated with soft-tissue injuries. Some studies also show accelerated recovery.[100] The benefits of proteolytic enzymes in DOMS are still yet to be proven in a randomized clinical trial. The mechanism of action of proteolytic enzyme is hypothesized to be that they work by degrading fibrin deposits, improving the drainage of debris and allow more oxygen and nutrients to reach the site. If this is in fact the case, there may be benefits to post-exercise recovery.

Branched Chain Amino Acids (BCAAs) — The BCAAs leucine, isoleucine and valine are found in muscle proteins. BCAAs are broken down in muscle during exercise. BCAA supplementation before exercise improves muscle recovery by decreasing the release of essential amino acid from exercising muscle. Evidence also exists to show BCAA supplementation just prior to exercise increases protein synthesis in skeletal muscle.[101] BCAA supplementation not

---

[99] Bryer, S. C., and Allan H. Goldfarb. "Effect of high dose vitamin C supplementation on muscle soreness, damage, function, and oxidative stress to eccentric exercise." International journal of sport nutrition and exercise metabolism 16.3 (2006): 270.

[100] Trickett P. Proteolytric enzymes in treatment of athletic injuries, Appl There 1964;6:647-652.

[101] Shimomura, Yoshiharu, et al. "Branched-chain amino acid supplementation before squat exercise and delayed-onset muscle soreness." *International journal of sport nutrition and exercise metabolism* 20.3 (2010): 236-244.

only attenuates muscle soreness, but also increases function specifically when consumed before exercise and three days after exercise.[102]

Taurine — Unlike the BCAAs discussed above, taurine is a nonessential amino acid because our bodies can produce it from methionine via cysteine with the help of vitamin B6. Taurine is present exclusively in animal products, especially meat and fish. It has a lot of functions throughout the body which are anti-inflammatory and antioxidative. Ra and colleagues divided 36 untrained male volunteers into four groups (BCAA vs. placebo vs. BCAA + Taurine vs. Taurine). Blood biochemical markers as well as subjective experience of DOMS were significantly reduced in the BCAA + Taurine group. The authors concluded supplemental taurine in combination with BCAA would be a useful way to attenuate DOMS and muscle damage caused by high intensity exercise.[103]

Sleep — Last but not least, good-quality sleep is restorative, and an important element in helping our body regenerate and repair. During sleep your body increases production of growth hormone. Everyone's "ideal" sleep duration is unique, but to be safe aim for eight to nine hours a night. Studies show that if you stay awake when you normally sleep there is no surge in growth hormone.[104] The good news is that once sleep is restored after periods of deprivation, extra hormone is released. But, just because your body can catch up does not mean you should make a habit out of late nights. Doing so will result in increased soreness and fewer muscle gains.

---

[102] Jackman, Sarah R. et al. "Branched-Chain Amino Acid Ingestion Can Ameliorate Soreness From Eccentric Exercise". Medicine & Science in Sports & Exercise 42.5 (2010): 962-970. Web.

[103] Ra, Song-Gyu, et al. "Additional effects of taurine on the benefits of BCAA intake for the delayed-onset muscle soreness and muscle damage induced by high-intensity eccentric exercise." *Taurine 8*. Springer New York, 2013. 179-187.

[104] Davidson, J. R., H. Moldofsky, and F. A. Lue. "Growth hormone and cortisol secretion in relation to sleep and wakefulness." *Journal of Psychiatry and Neuroscience* 16.2 (1991): 96.

Anti-Inflammatory Drugs

In the past non-steroidal anti-inflammatory drugs (NSAIDs) like ibuprofen were one of the few treatments for muscle pain. Personally, I use natural therapies when possible, as evidence shows the use of these over-the-counter painkillers to reduce muscle growth can cause damage to the liver with long-term use.[105]

Examples of powerful natural anti-inflammatories include curcumin, fish oil, spirulina, ginger, boswelia, resveratrol and alpha lipoic acid.

---

[105] Trappe, Todd A., et al. "Effect of ibuprofen and acetaminophen on postexercise muscle protein synthesis." *American Journal of Physiology-Endocrinology and Metabolism* 282.3 (2002): E551-E556.

CHAPTER FIFTEEN

Autoimmunity

AUTOIMMUNITY CAN BE DESCRIBED AS A CONDITION THAT DEVELOPS WHEN THE IMMUNE SYSTEM MISTAKENLY ATTACKS HEALTHY CELLS IN THE BODY. Autoimmunity can take on many different forms as it can affect any part of the body. For some, it results in hormone disruption, and for others, it can present as pain, fatigue, or even neurological changes. Despite a variety of clinical signs and symptoms, autoimmune diseases are a result of immune system changes that cause inflammation and damage.

What is most concerning with autoimmune disease is that the incidence rates are increasing worldwide by 4 to 7% every year. Notably, there has been the greatest increases in celiac disease, type 1 diabetes, and myasthenia gravis - a condition that causes rapid fatigue of the muscles. To date, according to The National Institutes of Health (NIH), up to 23.5 million Americans currently suffer from one or more autoimmune diseases. And, once you have one autoimmune disease, you are more likely to develop another.

What Causes Autoimmune Disease?

The development of autoimmune disease is multifactorial, meaning there is no singular cause. There are multiple variables linked to the onset of the condition including genetics, environmental toxins, stress and infectious causes. Some studies have shown that genetic predisposition accounts for only roughly 30% of all autoimmune diseases, leaving the remaining 70% as the result of environmental factors, like toxic chemicals, diet, infections, and gut dysbiosis. This is actually great news because it means that with early detection, in combination with dietary and lifestyle changes, we can identify, slow down, and even reverse autoimmune disease.

Foods and Toxic Chemicals Can Trigger Autoimmunity

Our immune system is filled with immune cells that stand guard defending our bodies against foreign materials like toxins and foods. A key class of immune cells are antigen presenting cells (APCs) which include macrophages and dendritic cells. These cells are triggered by foreign material and their job is to sound the alarm to the immune system that a suspicious particle has entered. This stimulates the immune system to produce cytokines and release them into circulation. Anti-inflammatory cytokines are released to stimulate the T-regulatory cells to monitor the reaction, while pro-inflammatory cytokines trigger inflammation and antibody production. The balance of two is critical, and imbalances cause autoimmunity.

The T-regulatory cells are like the bouncers who have the power to intervene in the process and stop the inflammatory immune reaction by developing tolerance. This is why we can consume foreign foods or be exposed to environmental allergens and not mount an immune reaction. However, if T-regulatory cells do not step up, then naive T cells will continue reacting and start to morph into TH1, TH17 and TFH cells. These immune cells can trigger autoimmune disease when the inflammation gets out of control, antibodies are produced, and tissues are damaged. It is the breakdown of immunological tolerance that leads to autoimmune responses that we see in the development of autoimmune disease.

When the body is healthy, the immune system is able to distinguish that yes, this cell is "me." However, there are toxic chemicals in our environment that enter into tissues and form bonds with healthy cells. This changes the structure and makes them unrecognizable to the immune system. This is where T cells bind to the cell they now don't recognize and call over their B cell friends to make antibodies beginning the attack on its own healthy tissues.

Literature exists showing that toxic chemicals and foods that can trigger autoimmune disease, yet little is done to prevent human exposure. Some of the chemicals include bisphenol A (BPA), mercury, asbestos, mycotoxins, trichloroethylene (TCE), benzoquinones, formaldehyde, ethylene oxide, penicillins, cigarette smoke, nail polish, sodium (salt), gluten, dairy, and glyphosate.[106] While it is unlikely that one exposure will cause autoimmunity, with genetic predisposition and multiple daily exposures, one can see how the risk of autoimmune disease is elevated.

Here are some examples of toxins and their relationship to autoimmunity:

- Nail polish contains halogenated compounds that can bind to mitochondrial proteins, changing their immunogenicity and inducing anti-mitochondrial antibodies.[107]
- Cigarette smoke and alcohol consumption are capable of modifying DNA methylation which results in changes in gene expression.[108]

---

[106] Rieger R, Gershwin ME. The X and why of xenobiotics in primary biliary cirrhosis. Journal of Autoimmunity. 2007;28(2):76-84.

[107] Bigazzi PE. Autoimmunity caused by xenobiotics. Toxicology. 1997;119(1):1-21.

[108] Machnik A, et al. Macrophages regulate salt-dependent volume and

- An excess uptake of salt can affect the innate immune system by interfering with macrophage function through TH-17 cells.[109,110]

- Drinking cow's milk may induce autoimmunity due to cross-reactivity of its albumin component with islet cell antigen-1 and beta cell surface protein.[111]

- A wheat-based diet induces not only TH1-type cytokine bias in the gut but also increased T-cell reactivity to gluten, with a higher frequency of diabetes.[105]

- Gluten increases zonulin levels (a marker of leaky gut) and the upregulation of genetically susceptible individuals may lead to autoimmune disease.[112]

- Glyphosate exposure has been linked to a non-exhaustive list of possible diseases which include autism, multiple sclerosis, type 1 diabetes, celiac disease, inflammatory bowel disease, and neuromyelitis optical.[113,114]

---

blood pressure by a vascular endothelial growth factor-C–dependent buffering mechanism. Nature Medicine. 2009;15:545-552.

[109] Cavallo MG, et al. Cell-mediated immune response to β casein in recent-onset insulin-dependent diabetes: implications for disease pathogenesis. Lancet. 1996;348(9032):926-928.

[110] Fairweather D, Rose, NR. Women and Autoimmune Diseases. Emerg Infect Dis. 2004 Nov; 10(11): 2005–2011.

[111] MacFarlane AJ, et al. A Type 1 Diabetes-related Protein from Wheat (Triticum aestivum) cDNA Clone of a Wheat Storage Globulin, Glb1, Linked to Islet Damage. J Bio Chem. 2003;278:54-63.

[112] Fasano, Alessio. "Zonulin, regulation of tight junctions, and autoimmune diseases." Annals of the New York Academy of Sciences 1258.1 (2012): 25-33.

[113] Samsel, Anthony, and Stephanie Seneff. "Glyphosate, pathways to modern diseases II: Celiac sprue and gluten intolerance." Interdisciplinary toxicology 6.4 (2013): 159-184.

[114] Samsel, Anthony, and Stephanie Seneff. "Glyphosate pathways to modern diseases VI: Prions, amyloidoses and autoimmune neurological

Microbes That Are Associated with Autoimmune Disease

Like toxic chemicals and foods, pathogens also have the ability to trigger autoimmune disease. Pathogenic infections, meaning microbes that have the ability to cause disease, are thought to stimulate autoimmune disease in four different ways: molecular mimicry, epitope spreading, dysregulation of immune homeostasis, and the bystander effect.

Molecular mimicry — Every cell in our body contains proteins that the immune system looks at to determine if it is self or non-self. Invading organisms are able to evade detection through molecular camouflage. Certain pathogens can develop epitopes of themselves that look exactly like epitopes of healthy human tissues which allows the pathogen to avoid immune detection and start to multiply within the cells. The issue is that if the immune system does recognize the pathogen and starts to produce antibodies, those same antibodies will also damage self-tissue because of the close resemblance.

Epitope spreading — Some pathogens are able to get into healthy cells and hijack the cell's machinery such that it produces proteins that favour the virus or bacteria. Eventually, these proteins force the cell to burst open and release the now multiple pathogens and their weapons throughout the body.

Immune dysregulation — This occurs when the immune system shifts and remains in an inflammatory phase that breeds autoimmune disease. When the body is healthy the T-regulatory cells (the referees) should shift the immune system from the inflammatory phase into an adaptive phase, where it begins to develop tolerance. Being forced to remain in the pro-inflammatory state is a breeding ground for autoimmune disease.

The bystander effect — When viruses, fungi, parasites, or bacteria infect healthy tissue, collateral damage is done to healthy non-

diseases." J. Biol. Phys. Chem 17 (2017): 8-32.

infected cells surrounding the area. This is because inflammation signals an influx of immune cells like natural killer cells to take care of the invaders. The immune system does a great job at attacking infected tissue but they are sloppy and often damage surrounding tissue. When healthy tissue is damaged, there can be miscommunication and continued attack on healthy tissues.

Pathogenic infections have been associated with a vast number of autoimmune diseases.[106,107] This table depicts some of the more common pathogen-associated autoimmune diseases.

AUTOIMMUNE DISEASE	ASSOCIATED PATHOGEN(S)
Rheumatic fever	*Streptococcus pyogenes*
Guillain-Barre syndrome	*Campylobacter jejuni*, Cytomegalovirus, Epstein-Barr virus
Type 1 diabetes mellitus	Coxsackie virus B4, Rubella virus, Cytomegalovirus
Lupus erythematosis	Epstein-Barr virus
Thyroid autoimmunity	*Yersinia enterocolitica*, Epstein-Barr virus, Parvovirus, Hepatitis C, Coxsackie virus
Rheumatoid arthritis	*Yersinia enterocolitica*, *Streptococcus pyogenes*, *Campylobacter jejuni*, *Klebsiella pneumoniae*, Hepatitis C, Epstein-Barr virus

Lyme disease	*Borrelia burgdorferi*
Multiple sclerosis	*Chlamydia pneumoniae*, Epstein-Barr, Human Herpes virus 6, Hepatitis B
Sjögren's syndrome	Epstein-Barr virus, Cytomegalovirus, Hepatitis B, Hepatitis C, Coxsackie virus B4, Human T-cell leukemia virus
Scleroderma	Cytomegalovirus
Myasthenia gravis	Herpes simplex virus, Hepatitis C
Primary biliary cirrhosis	*Escherichia coli*
Reiter's syndrome	*Chlamydia trachomatis, Shigella* species
Allergic encephalitis	Measles virus
Myocarditis	Coxsackie virus B3, Cytomegalovirus, *Chlamydia*
HTLV-associated myelopathy	Human T-cell leukemia virus

Microbial Diversity & Gut Dysbiosis

The gut microbiome needs to include a variety of healthy bacteria in order to thrive. Research shows that low microbial diversity in the gut is also associated with increased risk for autoimmune disease and increased incidence of infection.[108] A 2015 study showed that just one week of broad-spectrum antibiotics can negatively impact the gut microbiome, decreasing the microbial diversity for up to a years after the medications have left the system.[115] This study concluded that "clearly, even a single antibiotic treatment in healthy individuals contributes to the risk of resistance development and leads to long-lasting detrimental shifts in the gut microbiome."

The key to restoring gut biodiversity is to support the beneficial bacteria that reside in the gut, like *Bacteroides fragilis*, *Faecalibacterium prausnitzii*, *Akkermansia muciniphila*, *Bacillus* spores, and non-infectious *Clostridia* spp. These microbes can all help protect against autoimmune disease through the up-regulation of the T-regulatory system, suppression of TH-17, restoration of the intestinal mucus layer, and the reduction of systemic inflammation.[104] In this way, reconditioning the gut microbiome can help prevent and correct autoimmune responses within the body.

Summary

In summary, autoimmune disease develops from multiple triggers. Often a genetic predisposition exists, but many modifiable environmental triggers lead to the development and progression on autoimmunity. Ways to intervene and reduce the risk of autoimmunity include reducing toxic chemical exposure, dietary interventions as well as removing pathogenic infections, and supporting a healthy gut microbiome.

Environmental health solutions:

- Dramatically reduce your sodium intake

---

[115] Wischmeyer, Paul E. "Glutamine: role in gut protection in critical illness." Current Opinion in Clinical Nutrition & Metabolic Care 9.5 (2006): 607-612.

- Grow your own food when possible to minimize glyphosate exposure
- Consume prebiotic fibre
- Use natural household cleaners when possible
- Avoid skincare or cosmetics that aren't safe for human consumption
- Avoid dairy
- Limit or avoid antibiotic use unless absolutely necessary
- Avoid gluten and crops that use glyphosate for desiccation (corn, potatoes, barley, oats, etc.)

Gut health solutions:

- Eat a variety of fruit and vegetables to promote biodiversity in the gut
- Take *Bacillus* spores to help repair leaky gut and improve microbial diversity
- Avoid prolonged antimicrobial use when possible
- Keep fat intake below 30% of daily caloric intake to up-regulate the T-regulatory system and reduce the Firmicutes/Bacteroidetes ratio.
- Fast 14-16 hours daily (intermittent fasting) to promote increases in *Akkermansia muciniphila*.[116]
- Consume prebiotic fibres like xylooligosaccharies (XOS), fructooligosaccharides (FOS), and galactoligosaccharides (GOS) that feed only beneficial bacteria to improve microbial diversity. Kiwi contains these prebiotic fibres, but you must consume the entire kiwi.
- Supplement with gut healing herbs, IgG powder, L-glutamine, and nutrients like L-proline, L-serine, L-threonine and L-cysteine to repair leaky gut.[117]

---

[116] Vojdani A. A Potential Link between Environmental Triggers and Autoimmunity. Autoimmune Diseases. 2014;2014: Article ID 437231.

[117] Derrien, M., Belzer, C., & de Vos, W. M. (2015). *Akkermansia muciniphila* and its role in regulating host functions. Microbial Pathogenesis.

CHAPTER SIXTEEN

Mindset

WANT TO LEARN HOW TO LOVE YOURSELF?

I have an important question for you: *What will it take for you to become comfortable with who you are…as you are?*

We are not perfect, and some of us are less perfect than others. Have you ever had thoughts such as, "I am not as good as other people" or, "I am not where I want to be"?

These thoughts may arise because you don't like the way you look. Or, maybe there is something about your health, your behavior, or thinking patterns that you just don't like. Maybe you are dissatisfied with the way you feel. Maybe you don't like the circumstances of your life, your career, or the relationship you are in, and because of that you can't love yourself. This used to be me.

Let me tell you a secret: It is NOT always easy to love yourself…

I have always been insecure with my physical appearance. When I looked in the mirror there was always something I could nit-pick about. There was always something I didn't like, always something I could improve on or be better at. I was always criticizing and comparing myself to others.

This negative self-talk was perpetuating and hard to overcome.

If you are like me, it will take some inner work to realize you can be happy the way you are, despite any imperfections you may have.

To be honest, 99.9% of the time others don't judge you for your imperfections. Those judgments are loudest when they are coming from within YOU.

Consider this: everything has resonance or a vibration frequency, which is determined by the complex interaction of our thoughts, feelings, and behaviours. When you are comfortable in your own skin, other people will become "in-tune" with and accept that. Have you ever been around someone and just got a weird vibe from them? This is the law of resonance, or the law of attraction, working.

These laws determine precisely what it is you will attract in your life based on the resonance or frequency of the energy you are projecting. When you are constantly insecure with your own imperfections and you are expecting others to judge you for them, you are fulfilling your own prophecy. What you expect, you find.

Ask yourself right now: do you really not like yourself, all of you? Or, is it just an aspect?

If the answer is just an aspect, then think about how much time and energy you are spending on just this one aspect. Be truthful with yourself right now in this moment.

Ask yourself: "Is this imperfection within context of my entire life?"

Look at where you are, where you have been, and where you are going. If it is the case that this flaw is just a small aspect of you truly are, then realize it.

Also realize that you have the ability to control where you focus. If you are always magnifying your imperfections, then you are losing focus on all the good in your life.

I want you to make the decision right NOW. You have two choices.

Are you going to fix this imperfection or not?

If you can change it and wish to, then go for it. I am all about making your life objectively good. If you can't change it or don't want to, then you need to accept it. Accept your flaws and then shift your focus away. It is the constant focus and attention that is making you unhappy. Once you do this, you will be able start focusing on other areas of your life that are great!

Once you make this shift, you will notice that your little imperfections are insignificant in the context of all the other amazing things flourishing in your life.

I want you to start this exercise right now. I want you to commit to unconditionally loving yourself every day. I want you to believe in your heart that you are awesome (*because you are!*) I want you to stare at your reflection in the mirror and repeat to yourself everyday:

"I love and accept you, exactly as you are."

I want you to say this and really believe it. If negative thoughts or feelings arise, I want you to repeat the phrase again and again. You are more than just one trait you consider a flaw. You are more than your current or past personality or behavior. You are more and have so much to offer others.

If you think this exercise is silly or useless, or if you hesitate, I challenge you to ask yourself, "WHY?"

I also want you to consider this: if you don't love yourself, you cannot live a powerful life and serve others the way you want to.

Without loving yourself first, you cannot do good for others in the world. In fact, you may be harming people by thinking this way because the negativity you feel in your life is contagious. This hurt you feel travels into your relationships and every person you come in contact with.

While doing this exercise, you may begin to realize how critical and tough you are on yourself. You may realize how much time in your day is taken away from all the good in your life because you cannot see past the wall of imperfections.

There is good news. You can change, but you can also accept. Accept yourself in this moment as you are, but also continue to develop yourself. You can change so many aspects of yourself. In life you can go in any direction you want.

There are countless possibilities but right now accept who you are. Give yourself permission to accept yourself. It is a split-second decision to accept who you are as yourself. Only you are holding yourself back from making this split-second decision. Use this as a foundation every day to continue to become more and more amazing.

I will leave you with these final thoughts: you are not your body, you are not your imperfections, and you are not one specific problem you are facing in your life right now…

So, who are you? What if you could absolutely love yourself? What is holding you back?

Negative Self Beliefs Are Sabotaging Your Ability to Live a Life of Happiness

The opinion you have of yourself is the most important opinion that you have. Too many people do not realize that how they feel about themselves affects what is perceived by others around them. What happens is your negative self-beliefs, in turn, affect your relationships, your opportunities, and your overall life.

Too many people go around feeling wrong on the inside. Too many people do not like who they are. Instead they focus on their faults and their weaknesses, and they are constantly critical towards themselves. These are all negative self-beliefs.

That recording of everything they have done wrong is always playing in their minds... "You are not patient enough," "You blew your diet yesterday," "You are a bad parent," "You are still struggling with that addiction," "You should be ashamed of yourself." With all the noise in their minds, they wonder why they are not happy. The reason they are not happy is because of this war going on inside their heads. We are not meant to go through life feeling wrong on the inside.

Stop focusing on your faults.

Quit overanalyzing your weaknesses.

Stop beating yourself up because you are not who you thought you would be.

Here's the key thing to remember: you are not a finished product yet. **Life is about progress, not perfection**. I say this often but I believe it to be true: *"little by little, a little becomes a lot."*

We have to learn to enjoy the life we are in right now. Absolutely you have some weaknesses; we all do. There probably are some areas where you know you need to improve. But, being down on yourself is not going to help you do better.

Having that nagging feeling that is telling you, "you don't measure up" or "you'll never get it right" is not going to move you forward. You have to accept yourself right where you are, faults and all. The changes and results you want may not be happing as fast as you'd like them to, but you need to trust in the process and accept yourself where you are right now.

The problem with not liking yourself is you're the only person that you can never get away from. You can get away from your boss, your neighbor, even at times hide from your kids, but you can never get away from you. You are always with you. If you don't like you, life is going to be very miserable. Don't live your life being against yourself.

You may have some things wrong with you, but you have a lot more right with you.

You may have a long way to go, but if you look back, you will see how far you've already come.

Keep your flaws in perspective. Every person has something they are dealing with. Every person at some time had negative self-beliefs but the key is to invest in changing your perspective. Social media is full of "the show." You may see someone who looks further along than you are. They look like they have it all together; they are happy and enjoying their life. They are successful, their kids actually listen to them, and they are in perfect health. BUT, the reason they are not upset, the reason they are not down on themselves, is they have learned this principle and they enjoy where they are at right now.

Often we think, "I'm going feel good about myself as soon as I lose the 10 pounds, as soon as I break this addiction, as soon as I control my emotions, then I will get rid of the guilt, the heaviness."

What I am asking you to do today is to feel good about yourself right, where you are at. Recognize any negative self-beliefs you may have and reframe them into positives. If you don't understand this, you will go through life not liking yourself. This is because as soon as you overcome the weakness in the forefront of your mind, as soon as you cross that deficiency off your list, there will be something else you need to improve upon. It will be a never-ending cycle.

Identifying negative core beliefs about yourself is often enough to understand recurring problems in your life. Identifying core beliefs either about yourself, others, or your world can complete your understanding of why a situation is particularly challenging or distressing to you.

Try and recall an intense or stressful situation. Identify any "hot thoughts" or automatic thoughts that arise. End this exercise by thinking, "Is this true?" Write down some evidence to support the thought and evidence against the statement. Lastly, think of a more "balanced thought." The more you do this, the less power negative core believes will have, and you will begin to understand your reactions and emotions better.

Another exercise I want you to get in the habit of doing is affirmations. To do this, write down three positive aspects of you in the form of "I AM" statements. Keep these in a place where you will see them regularly, maybe on the bathroom mirror, beside your bed, or on the home screen of your phone. Look at them daily and remind yourself you are doing the best you can and your best is always enough.

View Challenges as OPPORTUNITIES.

When I'm working to improve my mindset, the first thing I do is consider everything that happens as an opportunity to learn. What I mean by this is that there are so many times in business or in life that things happen that we get down on. Maybe you don't hit your goal that month, or you get in an argument, or you get a bill that you weren't expecting.

What you need to think of is how can you shift that negativity into a thought that is more positive so you can see the situation as a learning experience. What can you learn from that situation? Aim to shift from a place of, "This sucks" to a place where you say, "Okay, what can I learn from this opportunity?"

Consider every event an opportunity to learn and grow, instead of seeing these events as such negative things. Do you already do this? If you don't, what are some ways that you track abundance into your life?

There is Enough Abundance for EVERYONE

If you're going to have the right mindset, you also need to recognize that there is more than enough abundance for everybody. There is more than enough for you, there is more than enough for me, and there is more than enough for everybody in this world to have all the money they want, all the love they all, all the health they want. *There is more than enough for all of us.*

So, there is no need for jealousy or anger towards other people when realistically, the more you focus on that negativity, the more you are going to attract negativity. Focus on the fact that there is more than enough to go around if you want to attract more of what you want, which is abundance.

Surround Yourself with People Who You Want to BE Like

The people who you hang out with will directly reflect what you attract and who you become. I am a firm believer that who you hang out with will directly reflect the person you are, and the person you will become.

Mindsets are contagious. So, if you hang out with people who have a "lack" mentality, who believe abundance doesn't happen and who have a negative outlook on life, that mindset will shift over to you, as much as you don't want it to. If you believe that there isn't enough of the good stuff in life for everyone to get what they need, you are firmly rooted in a "lack" mentality.

You are the sum of the five people you hang out with the most. Take a little bit of an inventory. There may be people who you are going to need to choose to not hangout with because of their lack mentality. Maybe you need to unfriend or unfollow them because of their contagious negativity. As you continue to grow as a person, make sure you are hanging out with people that you want to be like in order to attract abundance. Make sure you are surrounding yourself with people who have what you want, because mindsets are contagious.

Give More to Receive More

You also need to give more of what you want. The best way to attract abundance is to give more. I know most of you are probably thinking that this is so counterintuitive. If you have no money, would you want to give money to somebody? OR, why would you give something to somebody that you don't already have yourself?

The thing is, the more you give, the more you will attract. Next time you are in a store and they ask, "Do you want to round up your number to give to a certain charity?" or, "Do you want to donate to XYZ Foundation," just do it.

I cannot explain to you how much my mindset has shifted around giving. I love giving things to people. A big way for you to attract more abundance into your life is to give. What can you give to somebody? It doesn't have to be money. Maybe you volunteer your time, or you help feed a family, or you provide a toy to a child.

Live the Life You Want to Live in the Future NOW

Don't wait to live the life of your dreams. Live the life you want to live in the future now. So, envision where you want to be in 5 years and in 10 years. Think about what you will be doing when you reach your goals. How will you carry yourself? How will you speak? How will you run your daily routine?

And from the very beginning, live as if you are already this person! Treat yourself and your business as if have already achieved success. Shift your mindset to this. Live the life you want to live NOW. So how can you shift? Where do you want to be? Is that a level in your company? Is that becoming a mom? Is it retiring? Wherever you want to be, live it now.

What steps can you take NOW to be living that life? What steps does that take? And what is that you doing even 2 years from now that you can be doing now? Just think about it. And the more you live that life, the more you will create that abundance and believe that this is going to happen, the more it is going to come to you.

Know the Power of Affirmations:

My last mindset tip is to recognize the power of affirmations. The power of "I am" is to believe that whatever follows "I AM" will come to you. If you choose to start your morning with "I AM grateful" and "I AM blessed" and "I AM loved," then those things will be attracted into your life, and abundance is going to come for you. But, if you choose to live your life from a place of "I AM suffering" or "I AM not enough" or "I AM" whatever negative aspect comes to mind, that's going to come for you, too.

I challenge you today to write five affirmations that start with "I am…" that are positive. For example, write down, "I am successful," "I am enough," "I am loved," "I am grateful." Whatever your affirmations are, write them down and pin them on the front of your computer. I also want you to record these same affirmations into your phone in a voice note. Then, I want you to listen to you "I AM" affirmations at least five times a day. These thoughts need to become engrained in your mind so you are filled, beaming and bursting with positivity.

In Summary

1. Consider everything that happens in your life, positive or negative, to be an opportunity for growth.

2. Recognize that there is more than enough for everybody. Get rid of that lack mentality and stop believing that there isn't enough for you. There is enough for every single person reading to have abundance. There is enough abundance for everyone.

3. You are the sum of the five people you hang out with the most, so choose wisely. Choose to surround yourself with people you want to be like one day.

4. Give more to receive more, regardless of whether that is money, or food, or time. Whatever it is, give more to receive more.

5. Live the life you want to live NOW.

6. Know and use the power of affirmations. Write down five affirmations and also record them. Read and listen to them at least five times per day.

CONCLUSION

It has been a privilege to help clients and patients all over the world who are struggling to get back to their health. I have been incredibly blessed and am eternally grateful to have met so many amazing people along the way. I am also honored that you have taken the time to read this book and to hopefully have impacted your life in some beneficial way. From the time I started the Wild Side, I committed myself to inspiring, advocating and educating those who I feel have been left behind and even dismissed by the conventional medicine community. I was also determined to create a tribe of women who uplift and encourage one another to be the best version of themselves. Through the Wild Side Community Facebook Group, I feel we have accomplished this. Thank you.

I hope you come away from this book equally motivated to get back to your health naturally and commit yourself to living a life full of abundance, happiness, energy, and confidence. I would love to continue to help you on your healing journey, so please join our online community or visit us in clinical practice if that is possible for you. If I can leave you with my most valuable piece of health info that would be to have fun every day. Make the choice each day on how you will allow both yourself and others to make you feel. You have the power to think positive thoughts, attract abundance and provide your body with a quality foundation to live your best life.

~Aim for Progress Not Perfection

Breanne

APPENDIX

Supplements

HERE ARE LISTS OF SUPPLEMENTS THAT YOU MIGHT CONSIDER TAKING TO COMBAT SOME OF THE HORMONAL IMBALANCES LISTED IN THIS BOOK. To ensure that you take the right dosage and that your supplements don't have any adverse reactions to anything else you're taking, you should consult with a medical professional before taking them. To book an appointment directly with me to discuss your health and supplement needs, please visit my website at breannekallonen.com.

Liver Support Protocol
Homocysteine supreme
Detox Support Packs
NAC /Glutathione
Curcum- Evail
Paleo Cleanse
Magnesium Glycinate
Castor Oil Packs

Protocols for Optimizing Adrenals

Adrenotone Plus
Electrolyte synergy
Liposomal Vitamin C
B Supreme
Selenium
Magnesium Glycinate

Protocols for Optimizing Thyroid Hormones
T3 Release – Wild Side
Adrenal Thyroid Replete – Wild Side
AminoAcid Supreme
Megaspore
Castor Oil Packs

Protocol for Estrogen Dominance
Calcium D-glucarate
B Supreme
DIM-Evail
Curcum-Evail
Castor Oil Packs

Protocols for Brain Health
Brain Vitale
GPC Liquid
Neuro Mag
Curcum-Evail

Protocols for Mitochondria/Energy
Mito-NRG
Mito-PQQ
Curcum-Evail/ Resveratrol

Protocols for Gut
Betaine + Pepsin
Megaspore
NAC
GI Revive
Vitamin D
OmegAvail

Zinc Supreme
L-Glutamine

<u>Protocols for Blood Sugar Balance</u>
Metabolic Synergy
Berb Evail
OmegAvail Hi-Po
Sensitol

<u>Protocol for Menopause Support</u>
Femguard + Balance
Adrenotone Plus
Phosphatidyl Serine
DIM
Megaspore
Castor Oil Packs

<u>Protocol for Hair Growth</u>
HSN complex
Twice a day multi
AminoAcid Supreme
OmegAvail Fish Oil

<u>Protocol for Anxiety/Overwhelm</u>
Catecholacalm
PharmaGABA
Megaspore
OmegAvail Fish Oil

<u>Protocol for Anxiety/Overwhelm</u>
Catecholacalm
PharmaGABA
NeuroMag
Megaspore

<u>Best Protein Product</u>
PurePaleo Hydrolyzed Beef Protein

ADDITIONAL RESOURCES

THE FOLLOWING RESOURCES WILL HELP YOU APPLY WHAT YOU'VE LEARNED IN THIS BOOK.

Recommended Products

Wild Side Wellness Cookbook — http://breannekallonen.com/product/wild-side-cookbook/

Wild Side 10 Day Challenge - www.breannekallonen.com/challange

Wild Side Inner Circle Monthly Health Club - http://breannekallonen.com/innercircle

Supplements: wild-side-wellness.myshopify.com

WildSide Community Faccebook Group

www.facebook.com/groups/147861385855192

Natural Skin Care: AlumierMD use code BA357A5B

Body Fat analyzer: Bodymetrix

Probiotics: MegaSpore code: WildSide

Blue blocking glasses

Wild One Herbals by Lisa Marie Holmes

Relaxation Aids - Muse Meditation Made Easy

Water Filtration - AquaSmart, Santevia, Berkey

Toxin-Free Household cleaning

Essential oils – Doterra

Queen of Thrones Castor Oil Packs - Dr. Marisol, ND

Health Information

Cosmetic information and the dirty dozen — www. EWG.org
Seafood choices — www.seachoice.org
Macro calculators — myfitnesspal.com

Lab Testing

Genetic Testing

Genos Research — www.genos.co
23 and me — www.23andme.com
Youtrients — www.youtrients.me

Functional Medicine Testing

Hormone Testing — dutchtest.com
Stool testing: GI Map
Foodsensivity testing
Urinary Organic Acids - Genova
SIBO breath test

General Lab Tests

Complete blood count with differential (CBC with diff)
Thyroid Panel: TSH, free T3, free T4, reverse T3, thyroid antibodies, TBG
Serum ferritin
Vitamin D: 25 OH D3 and 1,25 OH vitamin D3
High-sensitive C-reactive protein
Homocysteine
Serum folate
B12
RBC magnesium

Laboratories

Diagnostic Solutions
Great Plains Laboratory
Doctors Data
Genova Diagnostics
Meridian Valley
RMA
Spectracell

ABOUT THE AUTHOR

B REANNE KALLONEN IS AN ALL-ENCOMPASSING FEMALE EMPOWERMENT COACH. She helps high-achieving women like you boost energy, lose fat, and increase confidence through balancing hormones so you can really show up in your business, careers, and adventures in life.

Breanne is a mom of two and holds an honors degree in Biomedical Sciences and a Doctor of Naturopathy Degree. Breanne is the creator of the Wild Side Wellness and owns two clinical practices in Saskatchewan and Ontario.

breannekallonen.com